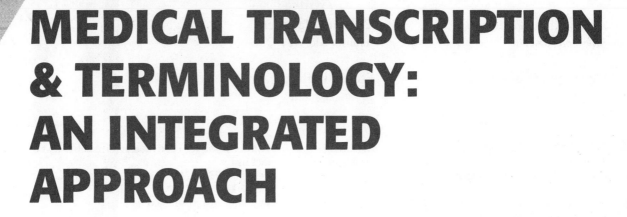

MEDICAL TRANSCRIPTION & TERMINOLOGY: AN INTEGRATED APPROACH

2nd Edition

Dr. Lois M. Burns, Professor
New York City College of Technology
The City University of New York
and
Dr. Florence C. Maloney, Professor Emerita
Kingsborough Community College
The City University of New York

THOMSON

DELMAR LEARNING™   Australia · Canada · Mexico · Singapore · Spain · United Kingdom · United States

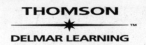

THOMSON

DELMAR LEARNING

Medical Transcription & Terminology: An Integrated Approach, 2nd Edition
Dr. Lois M. Burns and Dr. Florence C. Maloney

Executive Director
Health Care Business Unit:
William Brottmiller

Executive Editor:
Cathy L. Esperti

Acquisitions Editor:
Maureen Rosener

Developmental Editor:
Marjorie A. Bruce

Editorial Assistant:
Matthew Thouin

Executive Marketing Manager:
Dawn F. Gerrain

Channel Manager:
Jennifer McAvey

Project Editor:
Bryan Viggiani

Production Coordinator:
Cathy Ciardullo

Art and Design Coordinator:
Robert Plante

For permission to use material from the text or product, contact us by
Tel. (800) 730–2214
Fax (800) 730–2215
www.thomsonrights.com

Library of Congress Cataloging-in-Publication Data

ISBN: 0-7668-2692-9

NOTICE TO THE READER

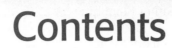

Contents

Acknowledgments

Our thanks are extended to the reviewers, the American Association for Medical Transcription, and especially to the numerous medical transcriptionists/medical language specialists in the field who contributed to this text.

This text is dedicated to all instructors of medical transcription and their students.

Reviewers

The authors would like to thank the following reviewers:

Selera Barnes
Charles County Public Schools
Charles County, MD

Laura Southard Durham, CMA
Forsyth Technical Community College
Winston-Salem, NC

Cheryl Hammel, RN, CMT
Memorial Hospital of Carbondale
Carbondale, IL

Patricia Kennedy, CMT
Pasco-Hernando Community College
New Port Richey, FL

Rosemary R. Lackey
The Andrews School
Oklahoma City, OK

Leo E. Nepon
St. Philip's College
San Antonio, TX

Suzanna M. Prosdocimo, CMT
Robert Wood Johnson University Hospital
Hamilton, NJ

Esther Storvold
Selkirk College
Trail, British Columbia, Canada

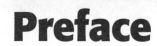

Preface

Medical Transcription & Terminology: An Integrated Approach, 2nd Edition, was developed to help learners enter the health care field as medical transcriptionists as quickly and easily as possible. The text format allows the learner to preview medical terminology, transcribe the dictated medical report, check the transcription to the text report, make needed corrections, and submit the corrected transcript to the instructor. One-third of the learner's class grade is related to the daily transcribed reports (the Instructor's Manual provides grading guidelines for these reports).

Then, as the learner becomes more confident and proficient in transcribing medical reports, the instructor can introduce weekly transcription tests. The tests should consist of terminology and punctuation previews and unfamiliar medical reports. The grades from these tests form the second third of the learner's grade.

The third component of the learner's class grade consists of grades from brief, weekly medical terminology quizzes.

ORGANIZATION

The learner has optimum opportunity through regular transcription classwork, supported by the text, to move through five types of medical reports: Section III, Consultation Reports; Section IV, History and Physical Examination Reports; Section V, Special Procedures Reports; Section VI, Operative Reports; and Section VII, Discharge Summary Reports. Each report is coded to one of twelve body systems.

Section I covers recent regulations and information relevant to document preparation and certification procedures. Sections II and VIII are new to the second edition. Section II, Miscellaneous Reports, includes other types of medical reports such as Outpatient Progress Reports, Pathology Reports, and OR Notes. In addition to reports coded to specific body systems, reports on neonate and psychiatric patients are also included. At the beginning of each section, each type of report covered in the section is described.

Section VIII, Challenge Reports, allows the instructor to assign reports for transcription with only terminology and punctuation cues provided. Learners will transcribe the report from the audiotapes and the instructor will compare the submitted transcripts to the reports in Section VIII of the Instructor's Manual. The reports are varied in length to accommodate individual learner abilities.

All reports are identified with the patient name and coded to a body system or medical specialty (as in neonate or psychiatric patients). The reports are arranged by length within the particular body system or medical specialty.

A new feature of the second edition is punctuation references. Each report in Section II contains a punctuation preview. Selected reports in Sections III through VII and all reports in Section VIII contain punctuation previews. Appendix C includes comprehensive punctuation references from *Grammar and Writing Skills for the Health Professional,* by Lorraine and Doreen Villemaire, Delmar Learning, 2001.

More illustrations were added to the second edition to enable learners to acquire a better understanding of body structure and disease, thus improving their ability to transcribe medical reports. Logs are provided throughout the text for learners to monitor their progress.

A CD-ROM is provided at the back of the text to provide medical terminology practice. *Delmar's Medical Terminology Flash!: Computerized Flashcards* contains more than 1,500 medical terms organized by body system. Flash! is a flashcard-type question-and-answer association program designed to help learners master correct spelling, definitions, and pronunciations of medical terms.

SUPPLEMENTS

The second edition of the text is accompanied by a set of six audiotapes containing practice medical reports for transcription. The same audio reports are also available for downloading from Delmar Learning's Internet site (www.delmarhealthcare.com/companions), at the Online Companion page for this title.

The Instructor's Manual contains guidelines for methods of study and evaluating learner performance. Fifty-one transcription tests with terminology previews are provided in the Manual and are correlated to Audiotape 6 (recorded test reports). Medical terminology short answer tests with answer keys are also included to provide additional learner practice.

The first edition of *Medical Transcription & Terminology: An Integrated Approach* received the Delta Pi Epsilon (National Honorary Professional Graduate Society in Business Education), Metro Chapter Author Award for Best Book Published in 1997 and is referenced by the American Association for Medical Transcription in its *Desk Companion 1998–2003* and was reviewed in the November–December 1999 issue of the *Journal of the American Association for Medical Transcription (JAAMT)*.

The authors wish abundant success and productivity to every learner in pursuit of a career in medical report transcription.

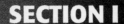

SECTION I

The Medical Transcription Profession

INTRODUCTION

The medical transcriptionist (MT) is a key member of the health care team and plays an integral role in preparing the descriptive information of the medical record, including consultations, history and physical examinations, operative reports, special procedures reports, and discharge summaries. Therefore, the medical transcriptionist is the vital link between the physician and the patient.

The American Association for Medical Transcription (AAMT) is the professional organization for the advancement of medical transcription, and for the education and development of medical transcriptionists as medical language specialists. AAMT has a membership of 8000. In 2000, AAMT had developed three distinct professional levels of model job descriptions for the medical transcriptionist (see Figure I-1). These are the most comprehensive descriptions of the duties and responsibilities available to guide and assist a medical transcriptionist in this profession.

EVOLUTION OF TRANSCRIPTION SKILLS

The medical secretary of the 1960s may have taken dictation from the physician in shorthand and transcribed it on the typewriter. Today's medical transcriptionist/medical language specialist may use sophisticated transcribing equipment and computer technology in preparing medical documents. Along with the new equipment, medical technological advances, medical procedures, medical instruments, and medical terminology, there are medical malpractice concerns. Medical transcription has become more specific, more diverse, and perhaps even more lengthy.

On a day-to-day basis, the medical transcriptionist is challenged by the number of doctors dictating with different dialects, additional terminology, and keeping familiar with the latest reference materials, for producing legible, accurate medical documents in a timely manner. The medical transcript is a legal document and subject to recall when there is litigation.

Medical transcriptionists must be proficient in English grammar, punctuation, spelling, and standards of style; must be fluent with medical terms; must be knowledgeable about anatomy, physiology, and pharmacology; must be able to comply with current government document preparation regulations; and must understand the legal implications of the practice of medicine.

CONFIDENTIALITY

Dedicated medical transcriptionists will recognize the importance of confidentiality. They must never discuss a patient's record or release information without a patient's written permission. Like the physician, they must never forget the portion of the *Hippocratic Oath* that states

> Whatever, in connection with my professional practice, or not in connection with it, I may see or hear in the lives of men which ought not to be spoken abroad, I will not divulge, as reckoning that all should be kept secret.

The proliferation of information and the increased use of the Internet are good reasons for patients to have concerns about confidentiality. In 1993, the drafting of the Health Insurance Portability and Accountability Act (HIPAA) legislation began. It represents the strongest federal confidentiality

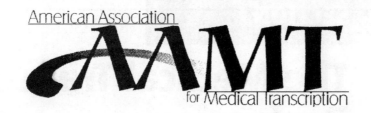

Medical Transcriptionist Job Descriptions
Results of a Benchmarking Analysis of MT Professional Levels

Professional Levels

In an independent benchmarking study of the medical transcription profession by the Hay Management Consultants (HayGroup), three distinct professional levels for medical transcriptionists were identified and described as presented below. The HayGroup is a worldwide human resources consulting firm with extensive expertise in work analysis and job measurement.

Compensation

Subsequent to this benchmark study of the job content levels of MTs, the HayGroup conducted a compensation survey, analyzing pay as it relates to these levels. (Hay's survey methodology complied with federal antitrust regulations regarding healthcare compensation surveys.) The results include information on transcription pay at the corporate level (healthcare organizations and MT businesses) and compensation for independent contractors. The data are further presented by geographic region, size of business, types of pay programs (pay for time worked and pay for production), and reward programs (benefits, etc.). The Hay report, "Compensation for Medical Transcriptionists," is contained in a 30-page booklet, available from AAMT for $40; $25 for AAMT members.

	Survey Benchmark Job Level		
	Professional Level 1	**Professional Level 2**	**Professional Level 3**
Position Summary	Medical language specialist who transcribes dictation by physicians and other healthcare providers in order to document patient care. The incumbent will likely need assistance to interpret dictation that is unclear or inconsistent, or make use of professional reference materials.	Medical language specialist who transcribes and interprets dictation by physicians and other healthcare providers in order to document patient care. The position is also routinely involved in research of questions and in the education of others involved with patient care documentation.	Medical language specialist whose expert depth and breadth of professional experience enables him or her to serve as a medical language resource to originators, coworkers, other healthcare providers, and/or students on a regular basis.
Nature of Work	An incumbent in this position is given assignments that are matched to his or her developing skill level, with the intention of increasing the depth and/or breadth of exposure. **OR** The nature of work performed (type of report or correspondence, medical specialty, originator) is repetitive or patterned, not requiring extensive depth and/or breadth of experience.	An incumbent in this position is given assignments that require a seasoned depth of knowledge in a medical specialty (or specialties). **OR** The incumbent is regularly given assignments that vary in report or correspondence type, originator, and specialty. Incumbents at this level are able to resolve nonroutine problems independently, or to assist in resolving complex or highly unusual problems.	An incumbent in this position routinely researches and resolves complex questions related to health information or related documentation. **AND/OR** Is involved in the formal teaching of those entering the profession or continuing their education in the profession. **AND/OR** Regularly uses extensive experience to interpret dictation that others are unable to clarify. Actual transcription of dictation is performed only occasionally, as efforts are usually focused in other categories of work.

Figure 1-1   AAMT Medical Transcriptionist Job Description

2   **SECTION I**

	Survey Benchmark Job Level		
	Professional Level 1	**Professional Level 2**	**Professional Level 3**
Knowledge, Skills, and Abilities	1. Basic knowledge of medical terminology, anatomy and physiology, disease processes, signs and symptoms, medications, and laboratory values. Knowledge of specialty (or specialties) as appropriate. 2. Knowledge of medical transcription guidelines and practices. 3. Proven skills in English usage, grammar, punctuation, style, and editing. 4. Ability to use designated professional reference materials. 5. Ability to operate word processing equipment, dictation and transcription equipment, and other equipment as specified. 6. Ability to work under pressure with time constraints. 7. Ability to concentrate. 8. Excellent listening skills. 9. Excellent eye, hand, and auditory coordination. 10. Ability to understand and apply relevant legal concepts (e.g., confidentiality).	1. Seasoned knowledge of medical terminology, anatomy and physiology, disease processes, signs and symptoms, medications, and laboratory values. In-depth or broad knowledge of a specialty (or specialties) as appropriate. 2. Knowledge of medical transcription guidelines and practices. 3. Excellent skills in English usage, grammar, punctuation, and style. 4. Ability to use an extensive array of professional reference materials. 5. Ability to operate word processing equipment, dictation and transcription equipment, and other equipment as specified, and to troubleshoot as necessary. 6. Ability to work independently with minimal or no supervision. 7. Ability to work under pressure with time constraints. 8. Ability to concentrate. 9. Excellent listening skills. 10. Excellent eye, hand, and auditory coordination. 11. Proven business skills (scheduling work, purchasing, client relations, billing). 12. Ability to understand and apply relevant legal concepts (e.g., confidentiality). 13. Certified medical transcriptionist (CMT) status preferred.	1. Recognized as possessing expert knowledge of medical terminology, anatomy and physiology, disease processes, signs and symptoms, medications, and laboratory values related to a specialty or specialties. 2. In-depth knowledge of medical transcription guidelines and practices. 3. Excellent skills in English usage, grammar, punctuation, and style. 4. Ability to use a vast array of professional reference materials, often in innovative ways. 5. Ability to educate others (one-on-one or group). 6. Excellent written and oral communication skills. 7. Ability to operate word processing equipment, dictation and transcription equipment, and other equipment as specified, and to troubleshoot as necessary. 8. Proven business skills (scheduling work, purchasing, client relations, billing). 9. Ability to understand and apply relevant legal concepts (e.g., confidentiality). 10. Certified medical transcriptionist (CMT) status preferred.

Reprinted with permission from the American Association for Medical Transcription, Modesto, California, USA

protection ever enacted. The Privacy Rule became effective on April 14, 2001. Entities that are impacted by this rule have two years within which to comply before penalties are imposed. The rules of this legislation were written by the secretary of the Department of Health and Human Services (HHS).

EDUCATION

Education is of prime importance to achievement of success in the profession. While many experienced transcriptionists received their training on the job, most of today's transcriptionists are receiving their training at technical colleges and institutes. Many colleges are offering associate degrees with medical secretarial/medical transcription specialties. These programs often include courses such as medical terminology, medical office procedures, medical coding, medical transcription, keyboarding, word processing, Business English, and anatomy and physiology. Some programs include an internship program where the student gains "on-the-job" experience in a medical specialty department within a hospital, medical facility, or physician's office.

CERTIFICATION

The transcriptionist, if eligible, may apply to take the two-part certification examination and, upon successful completion, may become a certified medical transcriptionist (CMT).

Some major content areas of Part I (multiple choice) of this exam are: medical terminology, English language and usage, anatomy and physiology, disease processes, health care record, and professional development. Part II of the exam is transcription. Candidates must pass Part I in order to register for Part II. For additional information, go to the web site at www.aamt.org and click on "Certification."

EMPLOYMENT OPPORTUNITIES

Medical transcriptionists have a variety of employment opportunities and may be employed within the hospital setting; in a physician's office, medical clinic, nursing home, research center, insurance company, or medical publishing company; or by a medical transcription service.

Medical transcription services may offer the medical transcriptionist an opportunity to work at home and may provide the equipment and delivery service. While working at home offers the transcriptionist flexibility and independence, the transcriptionist must maintain a medical reference library to ensure concise medical transcripts.

Opportunities exist for transcriptionists to work full-time, part-time, freelance at home, or for private clients.

PROFESSIONAL AFFILIATIONS

The American Association for Medical Transcription (AAMT) is a professional organization representing alliances with standard-setting organizations, governmental and regulatory agencies, and other professional medical associations and technical organizations. AAMT's representatives are out in the real world of health care and health care documentation.

Membership benefits include an AAMT Help Desk with access to professional MT staff by phone, E-mail, or fax, providing assistance with style, translation, and new terminology. (These benefits are for practitioner, student, postgraduate, and associate members only.)

Subscription to the *Journal of the American Association for Medical Transcription* (*JAAMT*) is included with membership. *JAAMT* is published bimonthly, and features timely columns and articles on industry trends. Also included with membership is the *AAMT Desk Companion,* a comprehensive guide to available medical resources.

AAMT members have the opportunity to attend local, state, regional, and national meetings. They may participate in workshops and attend lectures in the field; visit exhibits of new equipment and become acquainted with the latest reference materials; and network with medical transcriptionists, supervisors, health care services, and educators.

Professional Medical Affiliations

The American Medical Association (AMA) is the professional organization for physicians. It represents the interests of individual physicians who work within hospitals and other health care facilities.

The American Health Information Management Association (AHIMA) develops guidelines for patients' medical record information and patients' rights.

The Joint Commission on Accreditation of Healthcare Organizations (JCAHO) is a voluntary health care accreditation agency that requires standards for contents of medical records, complete medical reports, acceptable medical abbreviations, and time constraints for dictation and transcription of medical reports.

Other medical affiliations are:

- Computer-Based Patient Record Institute (CPRI)
- American Society for Testing and Materials (ASTM)
- Health Information Management Systems Society (HIMSS)

Medical Transcription Industry Alliance

The Medical Transcription Industry Alliance (MTIA) was incorporated in 1993. Today it is a 200-member nonprofit international trade association of transcription company owners actively participating in establishing uniform performance standards of professional practice for this industry. It provides a forum for industry representatives to exchange information among themselves, their strategic partners in health care, and the vendors who provide the industry with the technology to meet the demands of their clients.

Institute of Medicine

On March 1, 2001, the Institute of Medicine (IOM) released the final report of its Committee on the Quality of Healthcare in America entitled *Crossing the Quality Chasm: A New Health System for the 21st Century*. This report addresses health care quality issues, emphasizing the need for the elimination of handwritten clinical notes and recommending clear, complete, and more legible documentation of automated transcribed notes.

CAREER OUTLOOK

Excellent opportunities for personal growth and career enhancement are projected to increase for medical transcriptionists and medical office assistants who meet the profession's standards. Employment of medical transcriptionists is projected to grow faster than the average for all occupations through 2010 due to increasing demand for medical transcription services (*Occupational Outlook Handbook*, U.S. Department of Labor, 2002–2003).

The majority of MTs work in comfortable settings such as hospitals, physicians' offices, clinics, laboratories, medical libraries, government medical facilities, or at home. An increasing number of MTs telecommute from home-based offices as employees or subcontractors for hospitals and transcription services or as self-employed independent contractors.

Job opportunities should be the best for those who have earned an associate degree from a community college or vocational school or certification from the American Association for Medical Transcription.

MTs had median hourly earnings of $12.15 in 2000, with the middle 50 percent earning between $10.07 and $14.41 and the highest 10 percent earning more than $16.70 (ibid.)

Advancements in speech recognition technology are not projected to impact significantly the job market for MTs because of the need to review and edit drafts for accuracy. Skilled MTs will be in demand to identify and appropriately edit the inevitable errors created by speech recognition systems and to create a final document.

For information on a career as a medical transcriptionist, contact:

American Association for Medical Transcription
100 Sycamore Avenue
Modesto, CA 95354–0550
Phone: (209) 527-9620
FAX: (209) 527-9633
Web site: www.aamt.org   E-mail: aamt@aamt.org

State employment service offices can provide information about job openings for medical transcriptionists.

The authors congratulate you on your decision to acquire technical training for entry into the profession.

We wish you much success in your pursuit of a medical transcriptionist or medical office assistant career.

LEARNING MEDICAL TERMINOLOGY WITH MEDICAL TRANSCRIPTION

The theme for this text is learning by doing (and practicing) that which is done on the job. By learning medical terms as they appear in medical reports and relating them to the pathologies being treated, students will find that they are quickly motivated to learn more and to discover that the transcription of excellent medical reports is not only challenging, but rewarding as well.

By practicing transcription of medical reports and correspondence, students will absorb medical terminology and understand the diverse types of medical reports that exist. Students should consult a medical dictionary as part of their preparation and practice.

METHOD OF STUDY

The suggested method of study and transcription practice is outlined in Table I-1. An evaluation guide of students' performance is also presented in Appendix E.

FORMATTING

Employers require reports to be in a format specific to their requirements. Consequently, you will see some sections such as "IMPRESSIONS" indented and blocked to call attention to their importance. You will note also alternate acceptable forms of number usage. As report formatting becomes regulated as to format, some of these variations will disappear.

CODING OF MEDICAL REPORTS

Each medical report has an individual code for easy identification. The first group of letters indicates the type of report, the second group refers to a particular body system, and the third group contains the initials of the patient. The report number in that group follows the decimal.

For example: CONFEMJH.2

CON   CONSULTATION REPORT—type of report.
FEM   Female Reproductive—body system.
JH   Janet Holsley—name of patient.
.2   Second CONSULTATION REPORT in the Female Reproductive group.

TABLE I-1: TIPS FOR SUCCESSFUL MEDICAL TRANSCRIPTION PERFORMANCE

Throughout the Course

1. Study prefixes, suffixes, and word roots to learn how medical terms are formed. Use *FLASH* computerized flashcards (Delmar) for regular review.
2. Study anatomy illustrations and related terminology.
3. Consult punctuation and style guides for formatting medical reports and correspondence. (See Appendix C.)
4. Increase speed and accuracy of keyboarding skill.
5. Use a medical dictionary and appropriate medical reference sources to increase understanding of transcribed reports. (See Appendix D.)

For Classwork Transcription

6. *Preview highlighted medical terms in each report.* Use supplementary references as needed.
7. Listen to the tape to identify significant aspects of the report.
8. Transcribe the taped dictation to the best of your ability; use medical spell check, if available.
9. Print out a hard copy of the dictation on your word processor.
10. Proofread carefully, checking each word in the transcript against the transcript in the text. **Be sure to check your transcribed draft to the text transcript *AFTER* completing the medical document.**
11. Record the number of lines transcribed and the number of minutes to complete the transcription.
12. Make any revisions; submit the transcript to the instructor.

For Test Transcription

13. Preview medical terms provided by your instructor.
14. Steps 7 and 8 above.
15. Proofread your transcription; make needed revisions; print out a hard copy; submit transcript to the instructor.

Miscellaneous Reports

OVERVIEW

In this section the student will be transcribing medical reports of varying lengths, each of which contains a preview of medical terms and punctuation references keyed to the line in which the punctuation appears. The student should follow the format illustrated in the miscellaneous hospital reports.

Excerpts from the text, *Grammar and Writing Skills for the Health Professional* by Lorraine and Doreen Villemaire, Delmar Learning, 2001, are in Appendix C and should be consulted for punctuation rules cited in each preview.

INSTRUCTIONAL OBJECTIVES

In this chapter, the student will:

1. Transcribe miscellaneous hospital reports, including outpatient progress reports, pathology reports, and OR notes.
2. Learn terminology specific to each report relative to the gastrointestinal, integumentary, and musculoskeletal body systems.
3. Transcribe discharge summaries of the neonate with previews of relevant terms.
4. Transcribe consultation reports for psychiatric conditions with previews of relevant terms.
5. Reinforce understanding of the use of commas, hyphens, semicolons, apostrophes, and quotation marks.

REMINDERS: Preview highlighted medical terms and punctuation references in the report.
Listen to the tape to become familiar with it.
Transcribe the report inserting punctuation "cues."
Print out a hard copy.
Check carefully your transcribed report word by word to the text transcript.

THE TRANSCRIPT IN THE TEXT IS CHECKED <u>ONLY AFTER</u> YOU HAVE COMPLETED YOUR TRANSCRIPTION.

Record the number of lines transcribed and the number of minutes needed to complete the report.
Make corrections; submit the corrected transcript to your instructor.

MISCELLANEOUS REPORTS INDEX

	Patient Name	Code Name	Word Count
Outpatient Progress Reports			
GAS	David Browne	OPPRGASDB.1	75
GAS	Wubao Wang	OPPRGASWW.2	82
GAS	Guillermina Cortez	OPPRGASGC.3	90
GAS	Michael Bukarcevska	OPPRGASMB.4	102
GAS	Rachel Ng	OPPRGASRN.5	245
Pathology Reports			
GAS	Roger Stedman	PRGASRS.1	74
GAS	Viola Lares	PRGASVL.2	75
GAS	Aurelia Bhatia	PRGASAB.3	76
INT	Doris Wu	PRINTDW.4	120
MUS	Walter Podgoretz	PRMUSWP.5	154
OR Notes			
INT	Beulah Traymore	ORINTBT.1	101
INT	Katrina Derojas	ORINTKD.2	128
INT	Madeleine Deutschman	ORINTMD.3	185
Discharge Summaries			
NEO	Elizabeth Jones	DSNEOEJ.1	335
NEO	Kathleen Lucas	DSNEOKL.2	621
NEO	Edward Carson	DSNEOEC.3	768
Consultation Reports			
PSY	Catherine DeLeo	CONPSYCD.1	840
PSY	Joan McDonald	CONPSYJM.2	840

OPPRGASDB.1	David Browne	Terminology Preview
S/P		Status post.
villous adenoma		Villous—pertaining to villi with fine, hairlike extensions.
		Adenoma—a neoplasm of glandular epithelium.
anastomosis		Surgical connection of two tubular structures.
proctoscopy		Inspection of the rectum using a proctoscope.

PUNCTUATION REFERENCE

All punctuation references are keyed to the following text: Villemaire, Lorraine & Doreen. *Grammar and writing skills for the health professional.* New York: Delmar Thomson Learning, 2001. (Please see Chapter 9 in text and Appendix C.)

Line 8	hyphen—compound modifier, Rule 1

OUTPATIENT PROGRESS REPORT

1 Name: David Browne   Chart #:
2 Date: 5/15/–   Service: Colorectal

3 ## FOLLOWUP VISIT

4 Seven weeks **S/P** low anterior resection for a **villous adenoma** of
5 the rectum with no evidence of carcinoma. The patient is clinically
6 asymptomatic.

7 PHYSICAL EXAMINATION is unremarkable. The rectal examination
8 reveals a well-healed **anastomosis. Proctoscopy** confirms these findings.
9 The patient has healed his incision well.

10 DISPOSITION:
11 1. I will see the patient during office hours in four to
12   six months.

13 2. Followup should continue together with Dr. Winters.

14 _____
15   Albert E. Dolman, MD

16 cc: Dr. Winters
17   Dr. Dossier

18 AED/bk

19 d: 5/15/–   Word Count 75
20 t: 5/15/–   OPPRGASDB.1

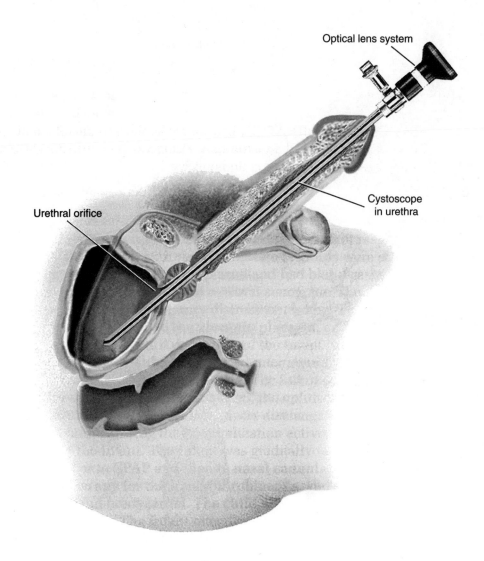

Optical lens system

Cystoscope in urethra

Urethral orifice

Cytoscopy

fistula	Fistula—an abnormal, tubelike passage from a normal cavity or tube to a free surface or to another cavity.
dissection	In surgical procedures, the cutting of parts for separation and study.
GD	Gastroduodenal.
cytoscopy	Examination of the bladder with a cystoscope.
retrograde IVP	A surgical procedure in which an endoscope is placed through the urethra into the urinary bladder; a catheter is then placed into the ureter for instillation of a contrast medium to visualize the renal pelvis and ureter.
rectourethral	Concerning the rectum and urethra.
myocutaneous	Pertaining to muscle and skin.

PUNCTUATION REFERENCES

| Line 7 | commas—series, Rule 1 |
| Line 10 | commas—series, Rule 1 |

OUTPATIENT PROGRESS REPORT

Name: Wubao Wang   Chart #:
Date: 4/19/–   Service: Colorectal

FOLLOWUP VISIT

Irrigations have demonstrated that the **fistula** remains open. The patient was advised that he will need a major **dissection** and separation of the rectum and prostatic urethra with a preoperative **GD** workup including **cystoscopy, retrograde IVP,** and urethrogram. The case was discussed with Dr. Sepali.

DISPOSITION:

1.   Admit May 1 for cystoscopy, retrograde IVP, and urethrogram on 5/1.

2.   Recovery and bowel prep on 5/2.

3.   Operation 5/3.

4.   Take down of **rectourethral** fistula with possible **myocutaneous** flap.

_____

William A. Blakely, MD

WAB/op

cc: Dr. Sepali
        Dr. Myers

d: 4/19/–   Word Count 82
t: 4/19/–   OPPRGASWW.2

gastroduodenal	Pertaining to the stomach and the duodenum.
NED	No evidence of disease.
asymptomatic	Without symptoms.
colostomy	A surgical opening of a portion of the colon through the abdominal wall to its outside surface.
edema	A local or generalized condition in which the body tisues contain an excessive amount of tissue fluid.

PUNCTUATION REFERENCES

Lines 4 and 5	commas—series, Rule 1
Line 7	semicolon—no conjunction, Rule 1
Line 9	hyphen—compound modifier, Rule 1

OUTPATIENT PROGRESS REPORT

1   Name: Guillermina Cortez   Chart #:
2   Date: 3/19/–   Service: Colorectal

3   ## FOLLOWUP VISIT

4   Two months S/P low anterior resection, multiple positive lymph
5   nodes, vascular invasion liver metastases complicated by rupture
6   of the **gastroduodenal** artery after an attempted dissection for
7   catheter placement. Clinically **NED; asymptomati**c.

8   PHYSICAL EXAMINATION is unremarkable. Rectal examination
9   reveals a very well-healed anastomosis. Her **colostomy** has no **edema**.
10   I will discuss with Dr. Lee the timing of her colostomy closure.
11   She is currently receiving Palauridine and 5-FU.

12   DISPOSITION:
13   Return visit will be based on closure.

14   _____
15   Warren C. Adler, MD

16   WCA/rt

17   d: 3/19/–   Word Count 90
18   t: 3/19/–   OPPRGASGC.3

erythromycin	An antibiotic effective orally against many gram-positive (Gram's method of staining to identify bacteria; retaining the color of the gentian violet stain) and some gram-negative (losing the stain and taking the color of the red counterstain in Gram's method of staining) organisms.
antihistamine(s)	A drug that opposes the action of histamine (a powerful stimulant of gastric secretion, a constrictor of bronchial smooth muscle, and a vasodilator that causes a fall in blood pressure).

PUNCTUATION REFERENCES

Line 6	comma—conjunction, Rule 3
Line 7	commas—series, Rule 1

OUTPATIENT PROGRESS REPORT

1 Name: Michael Bukarcevska   Chart #:
2 Date: 2/19/–   Service: Colorectal

FOLLOWUP VISIT

4 The patient has had what appears to be a very significant reaction
5 to **erythromycin**. He has a total body rash which has not responded
6 to **antihistamines**, and he has a marked swelling of his right arm
7 within the last 24 hours. The right forearm is warm, red, and has a
8 severe dermatitis. I have advised the patient to contact Dr. Jordan
9 regarding further treatment or referral. It is unwise to induce general
10 anesthesia for a colostomy closure tomorrow.

11 DISPOSITION:
12 1. The patient was rescheduled for admission February 28.
13   Operation to be on March 1.

14 2. Closure of colostomy pending resolution of the current problem.

15   _____
16   Walter Dodd, MD

17 WD/gh

18 d: 2/19/–   Word Count 102
19 t: 2/19/–   OPPRGASMB.4

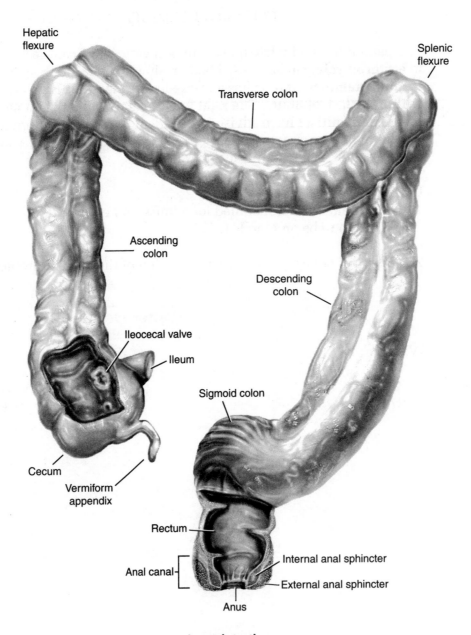

Large intestine

OPPRGASRN.5	Rachel Ng	Terminology Preview
colectomy		Excision of all or part of the colon.
ileocecal		Pertaining to the ileum and the cecum.
ileohypogastric		Concerning the ileum and the hypogastrium.
supraclavicular		Above the clavicle.
adenopathy		Glandular disease.

PUNCTUATION REFERENCES

Line 6	hyphen—compound modifier, Rule 1
Line 8	apostrophe—singular possessive, Rule 1
Line 11	hyphen—compound modifier, Rule 1
Line 15	comma—conjunction, Rule 3
Line 18	comma—conjunction, Rule 3
Lines 20 and 21	commas—series, Rule 1

OUTPATIENT PROGRESS REPORT

Name: Rachel Ng   Chart #:
Date: 6/19/–   Service: Colorectal

FOLLOWUP VISIT

Five months S/P total abdominal **colectomy** with ileorectal
anastomosis for a carcinoma of the colon situated 20 cm above
the **ileocecal** valve. There is biopsy-proven evidence of multiple
small liver metastases. At the time of the operation no evidence
of extra hepatic disease. The patient's recovery was complicated
by **ileohypogastric** nerve entrapment with severe pain delaying
any management until a recent block has eliminated the problem.
She now presents for her first post-operative visit and for discussions
of therapy.

PHYSICAL EXAMINATION reveals no **supraclavicular adenopathy**.
The liver is not enlarged to palpation or percussion. The incision is
well healed. The inguinal regions are normal, and there is evidence
of tenderness or discomfort on the left side. Rectal examination is
normal.

The patient was advised regarding the findings on the CT scan, and
the biopsy of the liver at the time of the operation. She is advised
regarding the options of treatment including no further treatment,
aggressive surgical resection, systemic chemotherapy, and/or regional
chemotherapy. The patient is advised for resection for the small
number of lesions and not for the multiple lesions evident in her
case. The patient is advised regarding the pros and cons of systemic
and regional chemotherapy. She is advised to review the options
and potential benefits and complications with an appropriate
medical oncologist. She agrees to the referral and is referred to
Dr. Clarissa Cohen for consultation.

_____

Matthew Hart, MD

MH/uw

cc: Dr. Clarissa Cohen

d: 6/19/–   Word Count 245
t: 6/19/–   OPPRGASRN.5

lipoma	A fatty tumor.
inguinal	Pertaining to the region of the groin.
formalin	An aqueous solution of 37% formaldehyde.

PATHOLOGY REPORT

1 PATHOLOGY NO.: 458 921
2 DATE: 11/21/—
3 CHART NO.: 67 32 10
4 NAME: Roger Stedman AGE: 61 Male
5 DEPARTMENT: Surgery MD: Dr. Maxwell Sander

6 TISSUE: **Lipoma** and sac of hernia

7 HISTORY: Recurrent right **inguinal** hernia.

8 Previous Operation: Repair of right inguinal hernia.

9 CLINICAL DIAGNOSIS: Repair of right inguinal hernia.

10 PATHOLOGICAL REPORT: Specimen received in 1 container in
11 **formalin** and is labeled lipoma and sac. Specimen consists of
12 two fragments of fat and soft tissue that measure $4 \times 3 \times 0.6$ cm
13 in aggregate. Representative sections submitted in 1 cassette.

14 MICROSCOPIC DIAGNOSIS: Lipomatous adipose tissue
15 and hernia sac.

16 _____
17 John M. Curran, MD
18 Pathologist

19 JMC/rt

20 d: 11/21/— Word Count 74
21 t: 11/21/— PRGASRS.1

PRGASVL.2	Viola Lares	Terminology Preview
polypoid		Like a polyp (a tumor with a pedicle).
dysplasia		Abnormal development of tissue.

PUNCTUATION REFERENCE

Line 12	quotation marks—words used in a special way

PATHOLOGY REPORT

1 PATHOLOGY NO.: RA92–189
2 DATE: 1/22/–
3 CHART NO.: 67 34 96
4 NAME: Viola Lares   AGE: 68 Female
5 DEPARTMENT: Surgery   MD: Dr. Mark Sanchez

6 TISSUE: Polypectomy—Colonic Polyp

7 HISTORY: Preop: Colonic Polyp—1 cm in diameter
8   at 27 cm from anal verge.

9   Postop: Colonic Polyp—Status Post—Colon
10   resection for cancer of the colon in '95.

11 PATHOLOGICAL REPORT: The specimen is received in formalin and
12 labeled "colonic polyp" consisting of a **polypoid** structure measuring
13 1 cm in diameter. Submitted in toto.

14 MICROSCOPIC EXAMINATION: 1 slide.

15 DIAGNOSIS: Colon at 27 cm (polypectomy). Tubular adenoma, with
16 mild superficial **dysplasia**.

17 _____
18 Sophie Todd, MD
19 Pathologist

20 ST/dn

21 d: 1/22/–   Word Count 75
22 t: 1/22/–   PRGASVL.2

serosa	A serous (producing or containing serum or a serumlike substance) membrane.
purulent	Containing pus.
suppurative	Producing or associated with generation of pus.
periappendicitis	Inflammation of surrounding tissue of the appendix.
mesoappendicitis	Inflammation of the middle of the appendix.

PATHOLOGY REPORT

1	PATHOLOGY NO.:	792 304
2	DATE:	12/20/–
3	CHART NO.:	56 84 20
4	NAME:	Aurelia Bhatia
5	DEPARTMENT:	Surgery

AGE: 15 Female
MD: Dr. Jane Brostman

6   TISSUE: Appendix

7   HISTORY: Right Lower Quadrant Pain

8   CLINICAL DIAGNOSIS: RLQ Pain

9   PATHOLOGICAL REPORT: The specimen is labeled appendix and
10 is received in formalin. The specimen consists of an appendix that
11 measures $6 \times 1 \times 0.5$ cm in greatest dimension. The **serosa** surface has
12 some white fibrinoid material attached to it and on a cross section.
13 Some **purulent** fibrinous material can also be seen. Representative
14 sections are submitted in 1 cassette.

15 DIAGNOSIS: Acute **suppurative** appendicitis with **periappendicitis**
16 and **mesoappendicitis**.

17   _____
18   Jon Tamurat, MD
19   Pathologist

20 JT/rp

21 d: 12/20/–   Word Count 76
22 t: 12/20/–   PRGASAB.3

PRINTDW.4	Doris Wu	Terminology Preview
fibroadipose		Containing fibrous and fatty tissue.
hyalinized		Refers to any alteration within cells or in the extracellular space that gives a homogeneous, glassy, pink appearance in reactive histological sections stained with hematoxylin and eosin.

PUNCTUATION REFERENCES

Line 10	apostrophe—singular possessive, Rule 1
Lines 10, 11	quotation marks—words used in a special way
Line 15	hyphen—compound words, Rule 1

PATHOLOGY REPORT

1	PATHOLOGY NO.:	963 354
2	DATE:	6/29/–
3	ACCESSION NO.:	36 20 18
4	NAME:	Doris Wu AGE: 68 Female
5	DEPARTMENT:	Ambulatory Surgery MD: Dr. Jonathan Elliot

6 ADMITTING DIAGNOSIS: Right breast mass.

7 CLINICAL DIAGNOSIS: Right breast mass.

8 TISSUE SUBMITTED: Right breast mass F/S.

9 GROSS: The specimen is received in the fresh state (frozen),
10 labeled with the patient's name and accession number as "RIGHT
11 BREAST MASS" and consists of an irregular portion of **fibroadipose**
12 breast tissue, 3.0 × 1.5 × 1 cm in greatest dimensions. No specimen
13 radiograph is received. No skin is received. There is a sharply
14 circumscribed rubbery mass 1 × 0.5 × 0.5 cm in greatest dimensions
15 with a gray-tan, slightly bulging cut surface. The entire margin is
16 inked in black. Representative sections submitted in 3 cassettes.

17 FROZEN SECTION DIAGNOSIS: Right breast biopsy **hyalinized**
18 fibroadenoma.

19 _____

20   Elizabeth M. Dodd, MD

21 EMD/gn

22 d: 6/29/–   Word Count 120
23 t: 6/29/–   PRINTDW.4

PRMUSWP.5	Walter Podgoretz	Terminology Preview
R/O		Rule out.
phenotypic		Refers to expression of genes present in an individual.
monoclonal		Arising from a single cell.

PUNCTUATION REFERENCES

Line 15	comma—conjunction, Rule 3
Line 22	apostrophe—singular possessive, Rule 1
Line 22	hyphen—with a prefix added to a word with a capital letter, Rule 3
	hyphen—with a single letter joined to a noun
Line 22	commas—appositive, Rule 7

PATHOLOGY REPORT

1   PATHOLOGY NO.:   329 486
2   DATE: 7/27/–
3   CHART NO.:   74 39 16
4   NAME: Walter Podgoretz   AGE: 51 Male
5   DEPARTMENT: Surgery   MD: Dr. Harry Saviou

6   TISSUE: Lesion of (L) shoulder. Frozen Section Diagnosis:
7   Skin: Atypical lymphoid infiltrate. Tissue sent out
8   for lymphoma workup.

9   HISTORY: Non-Hodgkin's lymphoma—S/P bone marrow transplant.

10   CLINICAL DIAGNOSIS: **R/O** lymphoma.

11   PATHOLOGICAL REPORT: The specimen is labeled lesion of (L)
12   shoulder and is received for frozen section diagnosis. The
13   specimen consists of a single irregular fragment of pink-tan soft
14   tissue measuring 2.3 x 1 x 0.5 cm in greatest dimension. Part of
15   the specimen is being sent out for lymphoma workup, and the rest
16   of the tissue is submitted for permanent sections in cassettes FS
17   and A1.

18   MICROSCOPIC DIAGNOSIS: 9593
19   The skin and subcutaneous tissue showed atypical lymphoid
20   aggregates of dermis and subcutaneous tissue. Lymphoid **phenotypic**
21   studies revealed Kappa **monoclonal** reactivity. These findings
22   indicate non-Hodgkin's malignant lymphoma, B-cell type, involving
23   skin and subcutaneous tissue. Evaluation of lymphoma subtype
24   cannot be properly done on the specimen received due to squeezing
25   artifact. Please correlate with previous slides showing lymphoma.

26
27   Barry D. Limguangco, MD

28   BDL/al

29   d: 7/27/–   Word Count 154
30   t: 7/27/–   PRMUSWP.5

ORINTBT.1	Beulah Traymore	Terminology Preview
infiltrating		Process of a substance passing into and being deposited within the substance of a cell, tissue, or organ.
cGy		Centigray.
iridium		A white, hard metallic element.

PUNCTUATION REFERENCES

Line 8	semicolon—one independent clause in a compound sentence contains a comma
Line 8	comma—introductory, Rule 7

OR NOTE

1 DATE: 5/1/–
2 PATIENT NAME: Beulah Traymore   DOB: 2/14/27
3 CHART NO.:   85 34 10
4 DEPARTMENT: Radiation Oncology

5 Patient has an **infiltrating** duct cell carcinoma of the right
6 upper inner quadrant of the breast. She received external
7 radiation therapy of 4500 **cGy**. She was brought to the operating
8 room; and under mammography guidance, the tumor bed was
9 implanted using 8 needles which were replaced by 8 ribbons. These
10 ribbons were secured later by buttons to the chest wall. The patient
11 will be brought down later to the department of radiation therapy
12 for simulation with dummy sources which will be replaced later with
13 radioactive **iridium**. The dose to be delivered will be 1600 cGy to the
14 tumor bed. The patient tolerated the procedure well.

15 _____
16   Janice R. Dolan, MD

17 JRD/ut

18 d: 5/1/–   Word Count 101
19 t: 5/1/–   ORINTBT.1

| interstitial | | Between the spaces within an organ or tissue. |

PUNCTUATION REFERENCE

Line 11   comma—introductory, Rule 7

OR NOTE

1   DATE: 7/17/–
2   PATIENT NAME: Katrina Derojas   DOB: 3/13/29
3   CHART NO.:   78 35 11
4   DEPARTMENT: Radiation Oncology

5   This patient has an infiltrating duct cell carcinoma of the left
6   upper outer quadrant of the breast. She had excisional biopsy and
7   lymph node dissection. The tumor was followed by external
8   radiation therapy and received 4500 cGy. The patient tolerated
9   the procedure very well. She was admitted for her boost to the
10   tumor bed using **interstitial** iridium implants to deliver 1600 cGy.
11   Under general anesthesia and with mammography guidance, the
12   patient had the left upper inner quadrant of the left breast implanted
13   using 6 ribbons. These ribbons were then secured with buttons. The
14   patient will be brought down to the department of radiation therapy
15   for simulation and computerized treatment planning. Loading will
16   be done with radioactive iridium to deliver 1600 cGy to the tumor
17   bed.

18   _____
19   Robert D. Whelan, MD

20   RDW/ad

21   d: 7/17/–   Word Count 128
22   t: 7/17/–   ORINTKD.2

fornices		The anterior and posterior spaces into which the upper vagina is divided. These recesses are formed by the protrusion of the cervix uteri into the vagina.
os		Mouth, opening.
necrotic		Death of a portion of tissue.

PUNCTUATION REFERENCES

Line 5	hyphen—prefix added to word with a capital letter, Rule 3
Line 9	comma—conjunction, Rule 3
Line 16	comma—conjunction, Rule 3
Line 17	comma—introductory, Rule 7
Line 19	comma—conjunction, Rule 3
Line 20	comma—conjunction, Rule 3

OR NOTE

1	DATE:	8/30/—	
2	PATIENT NAME:	Madeleine Deutschman	DOB: 4/25/31
3	CHART NO.:	29 03 74	
4	DEPARTMENT:	Radiation Oncology	

5 This patient is known to have non-Hodgkin's lymphoma for about
6 ten years and was treated with chemotherapy under the care of Dr.
7 Bradley. Several weeks ago she started to have vaginal bleeding
8 and a change in bowel habits. She was found to have a large
9 lesion in the vagina. A biopsy was performed, and it showed a
10 malignant tumor which could be lymphoma or carcinoma. This
11 patient also has lung metastasis. She was started on radiation
12 therapy to the pelvis and received 5000 cGy with an excellent
13 response. The tumor completely disappeared. She was brought to
14 the OR under general anesthesia. A pelvic examination was
15 performed together with Dr. Johnson. The vagina was completely
16 free of tumor except in the **fornices**, and the external **os** was
17 **necrotic**. In the fornices, there were about 1 cm of nodules on
18 each side which are highly consistent with malignancy. The canal
19 was dilated, and the uterus sounded to 9 cm. Fletcher applicators
20 were inserted, and the vagina was packed. The vulva was secured
21 and sutured by Dr. Johnson. The patient will be brought down to
22 the department of radiation therapy for loading with radioactive
23 cesium.

24 _____
25 Virginia Carr, MD

26 VC/mv

27 d: 8/30/—   Word Count 185
28 t: 8/30/—   ORINTMD.3

gravida	A pregnant woman.
para	A woman who has produced a viable infant weighing at least 500 g or of more than 20 weeks' gestation regardless of whether the infant was alive at birth.
dexamethasone	A synthetic glucocorticosteroid drug.
NICU	Neonate Intensive Care Unit.
IV	Intravenous. Injection into a vein.
bronchopulmonary dysplasia	An iatrogenic (related to any adverse mental or physical condition induced in a patient through the effects of treatment by a physician or surgeon) chronic lung disease that develops in premature infants after a period of intensive respiratory therapy.
hyperbilirubinemia	An excessive amount of bilirubin in the blood. In newborns, high levels of bilirubin may be caused by rapid destruction of red blood cells by prenatal use of certain therapeutic drugs or intrauterine viral infection.
apnea of prematurity	A condition of the immature newborn marked by repeated episodes of apnea lasting longer than 20 seconds.
sepsis	Spread of an infection from its initial site to the bloodstream.

PUNCTUATION REFERENCES

Line 3	hyphens—compound modifier, Rule 1
Lines 3 and 4	commas—series, Rule 1
Line 6	comma—introductory, Rule 7
Line 7	comma—introductory, Rule 7
Line 9	apostrophe—plural possessive, Rule 2
Line 10	comma—introductory, Rule 7
Line 17	comma—introductory, Rule 7
Line 17	commas—series, Rule 1
Line 19	comma—conjunction, Rule 3

PUNCTUATION REFERENCES (continued)

Line 20	comma—introductory, Rule 7
Line 21	comma—introductory, Rule 7
Line 22	commas—series, Rule 1
Line 24	comma—introductory, Rule 7
Line 26	hyphen—compound modifier, Rule 1
Line 28	commas—series, Rule 1
Line 32	hyphen—compound modifier, Rule 1
Lines 32–35	commas—series, Rule 1

| 1 | PATIENT: Elizabeth Jones | ADMITTED: 9/26/– |
| 2 | CHART #: | DISCHARGED: 11/19/– |

3 HISTORY/LAB: This infant was born on 09/26/– to a 30-year-old,
4 **gravida** II, **para** 1 female, with a last menstrual period of 3/22/–
5 estimated date of confinement 2/29/–. The mother had been followed
6 regularly during her pregnancy. However, she did develop preterm la-
7 bor necessitating early hospitalization. At that time,
8 the mother was placed on antibiotics and **dexamethasone** and
9 delivered at approximately 26 weeks' gestation. At the time of
10 delivery, the membranes ruptured spontaneously and fluid was
11 clear. The infant had an Apgar score of 5 and 8 at 1 and 5 minutes
12 respectively. The infant required intubation in the delivery room
13 and was then transferred to the **NICU**. On admission, weight was
14 1159 grams, length 38.5 cm, head circumference 25.5 cm, chest
15 circumference 26 cm. Assessment was 26 weeks' gestation.

16 COURSE/CONDITION ON DISCHARGE/DISPOSITION: At the
17 time of admission the infant had respiratory distress, was intubated,
18 and required Survanta. The infant was placed on **IV** fluids and
19 antibiotics, and appropriate blood work was done. During the
20 hospitalization, the infant improved with regard to the respiratory
21 distress. However, the infant developed **bronchopulmonary**
22 **dysplasia, hyperbilirubinemia,** and **apnea of prematurity**. The
23 infant was placed on the appropriate medications and improved
24 steadily. Her weight increased gradually. During the hospitalization,
25 the infant was evaluated by Dr. Lally of Ophthalmology who will
26 follow up on an out-patient basis.

27 The infant was discharged home on 11/19/–. She had had a hearing
28 test, eye examination as stated, and was going to receive home
29 physical therapy three times a week. She was on Fer In Sol drops
30 and was feeding on Neosure and breast milk. The overall prognosis
31 was guarded to good.

32 FINAL DIAGNOSIS: Preterm, 26-week female infant, appropriate
33 for gestational age, apnea of prematurity, anemia, respiratory
34 distress syndrome, bronchopulmonary dysplasia, hyperbili-
35 rubinemia, and presumed **sepsis**.

36 _____
37 John Cira, MD

38 JC/vs

39 d: 11/19/–
40 t: 11/19/–

Word Count 335
DSNEOEJ.1

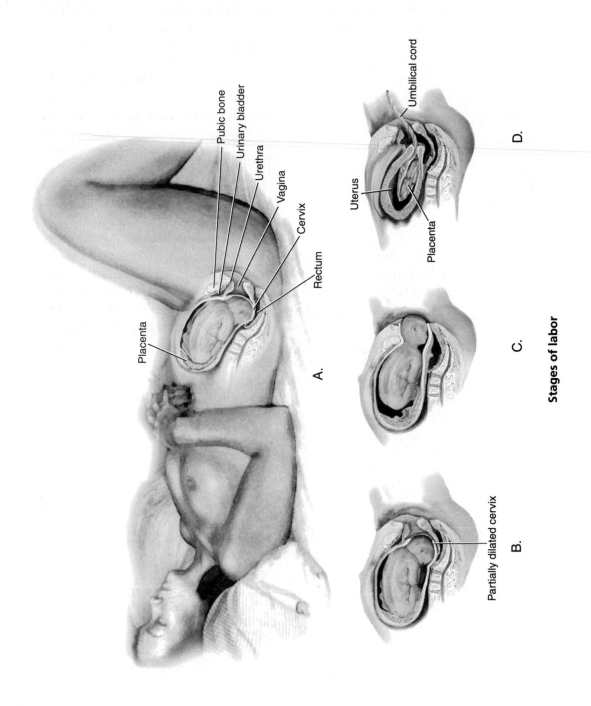

Pubic bone

Urinary bladder

Urethra

Vagina

Cervix

Rectum

Placenta

A.

Umbilical cord

Uterus

Placenta

D.

C.

Partially dilated cervix

B.

Stages of labor

abruptio placenta	Premature detachment of normally situated placenta after the 20th week of gestation.
weaned	The slow discontinuation of ventilatory support therapy.
CPAP	Continuous positive airway pressure.
nasal cannula	Tubing used to deliver oxygen at levels from 1 to 6 L/min.
phototherapy	The use of light to treat newborns.
hyperalimentation	The enteral and parenteral infusion of a solution that contains sufficient amino acids, glucose, fatty acids, electrolytes, vitamins, and minerals to sustain life, maintain normal growth and development, and provide for needed tissue repair.
patent ductus arteriosis	Persistence of a communication between the main pulmonary artery and the aorta, after birth.

PUNCTUATION REFERENCES

Line 4	commas—series, Rule 1
Line 4	hyphens—compound modifier, Rule 1
Line 7	comma—introductory, Rule 7
Line 8	apostrophe—plural possessive, Rule 2
Line 8	comma—conjunction, Rule 3
Line 10	commas—series, Rule 1
Line 12	apostrophe—singular possessive, Rule 1
Line 14	apostrophe—plural possessive, Rule 2
Line 15	commas—series, Rule 1
Line 17	comma—conjunction, Rule 3
Line 22	comma—conjunction, Rule 3
Lines 24 and 25	commas—series, Rule 1
Line 26	commas—appositive, Rule 7
Line 40	comma—introductory, Rule 7

PUNCTUATION REFERENCES (continued)

Line 44	commas—appositive, Rule 7
Line 49	hyphen—compound modifier, Rule 1
Line 50	hyphen—compound modifier, Rule 1
Line 50	comma—introductory, Rule 7
Line 51	apostrophe—singular possessive, Rule 1
Lines 51 and 52	commas—series, Rule 1
Line 55	comma—introductory, Rule 7
Line 59	hyphen—compound modifier, Rule 1
Lines 59–61	commas—series, Rule 1

| 1 | PATIENT: Kathleen Lucas | ADMITTED: 2/24/– |
| 2 | CHART #: | DISCHARGED: 5/12/– |

HISTORY AND PHYSICAL/LAB:

Baby Lucas was born on 2/24/– to a gravida 1, para 0, 33-year-old female who had a last menstrual period of 8/24/–. Her estimated date of confinement was 6/1/–. The mother had been followed during her pregnancy. At the time of delivery, the mother was approximately 25 weeks' gestation, and there had been fetal bradycardia on the tracing. The infant delivered having an Apgar score of 1, 5, and 7 at 1, 5, and 10 minutes respectively. The infant was attended to by the neonatal team in the delivery room and immediately brought to the St. Malachy's Hospital neonatal intensive care unit. Physical assessment at that time revealed the infant to be 25 weeks + 4 to 5 days' gestation with a head circumference of 25 cm, length of 36 cm, weight of 1500 grams.

COURSE/CONDITION ON DISCHARGE/DISPOSITION:

The infant was intubated and placed on an infant respirator, and antibiotics along with the appropriate IV fluids were started. The infant had umbilical lines placed and had blood gases followed along with chest x-ray and cerebral sonogram. The x-rays were consistent with respiratory distress syndrome. The blood counts were followed due to the **abruptio placenta**, and antibiotics were continued until negative and the infant had improved adequately. The infant developed pneumonia, apnea, bradycardia, hyperbilirubinemia, and anemia. The infant was followed during the hospitalization by Dr. Salerno, the ophthalmologist, who was scheduled to follow the baby upon discharge home from the hospital. The parents during the hospitalization actively participated in the care of the infant. The infant was gradually **weaned** from the respirator to **CPAP** and then to **nasal cannula**. The infant received **phototherapy** for the hyperbilirubinemia, and therapies for the apneas and bradycardia. The child also received antibiotics for eye drainage. The infant overall was weaned initially from the **hyperalimentation** to oral feedings. She was then able to take adequate intake by oral route and the IV was discontinued. The infant was also evaluated by the pediatric cardiologist and received Indocin for **patent ductus arteriosis** and numerous courses of antibiotics for suspected sepsis. The infant was monitored with electrolytes and blood counts regularly. The infant did have chronic changes in the lung taking place. However, the infant improved significantly enough gradually that we were able to send the infant home to be followed on an out-patient basis by the multiple consultants as well as by the pediatrician. The infant on the day of

44   discharge, May 12,–, was scheduled to see the private pediatrician in
45   approximately 4 to 5 days. She was scheduled to be followed
46   up by ophthalmology as stated above and by the gastroenterology
47   team for possible reflux and cardiology if any further complications
48   occurred. The prognosis was guarded to good. The parents were
49   instructed in care of a high-risk premature infant and were scheduled
50   for high-risk followup also. On the day of discharge, the physical
51   exam revealed the baby's weight to be 2265 grams, length 45 cm,
52   head circumference 33 cm, chest circumference 29 cm. The infant
53   had a regular rhythm with no murmurs. The abdomen was soft with
54   no masses. There was good range of motion of the extremities.
55   Neurologically, the infant had been evaluated and followed by
56   physical therapy and appeared to be doing well for the correct age.
57   The prognosis is guarded to good.

58   FINAL DIAGNOSIS:
59   Severe preterm 25-week gestation female infant, respiratory distress
60   syndrome, abruptio placenta, apnea, bradycardia, hyperbilirubine-
61   mia, anemia, presumed sepsis, pneumonia, and prematurity.

62   _____
63   Michael Estabrook, MD

64   ME/vs

65   d: 5/12/–   Word Count 621
66   t: 5/12/–   DSNEOKL.2

DSNEOEC.3	Edward Carson	Terminology Preview
VDRL		Venereal Disease Research Laboratory (test).
polyhydramnios		An excess of amniotic fluid in the bag of waters in pregnancy.
tachypneic		Pertaining to abnormal rapidity of respiration.
LGA		Large for gestational age.
TTN		Transient tachypnea of newborn.
tachycardia		An abnormal rapidity of heart action.
EKG		Electrocardiogram. A record of the electrical activity of the heart.
supraventricular		Located above the heart ventricle.
adenosine		A nucleotide containing adenine and ribose.
dilatation		Expansion.
myocardium		Middle layers of the walls of the heart composed of cardiac muscle.
Q-T		Electrocardiographic interval from the beginning of the QRS complex to the end of the T wave.
transient		Not lasting, of brief duration.
n.p.o.		Nothing by mouth.
H&H		Hemoglobin and hematocrit.
Enterovirus		A group of viruses that originally included poliovirus, coxsackievirus, and ECHO virus, which infected the human gastrointestinal tract.
q8h		Every 8 hours.
SIDS		Sudden Infant Death Syndrome.

PUNCTUATION REFERENCES

Line 5	comma—dates, Rule 4
Line 6	comma—introductory, Rule 7
Line 6	hyphen—compound modifier, Rule 1
Line 6	hyphen—adjective form, Rule 4
Line 6	comma—conjunction, Rule 3
Line 7	hyphen—with a single letter joined to a noun

Line 8	hyphens—compound modifier, Rule 1
Lines 8–9	commas—series, Rule 1
Line 11	commas—series, Rule 1
Line 13	comma—introductory, Rule 7
Lines 7, 18	commas—series, Rule 1
Line 18	comma—introductory, Rule 7
Line 20	hyphen—compound modifier, Rule 1
Line 21	comma—dates, Rule 4
Line 25	apostrophe—singular possessive
Line 25	comma—dates, Rule 4
Line 29	comma—introductory, Rule 7
Line 37	comma—introductory, Rule 7
Line 40	comma—introductory, Rule 7
Line 41	hyphen—compound modifier, Rule 1
Line 44	comma—introductory, Rule 7
Line 50	comma—introductory, Rule 7
Line 52	apostrophe—singular possessive
Line 54	commas—nonessential phrase, Rule 8
Line 57	comma—introductory, Rule 7
Line 58	semicolon—one independent clause in a compound sentence contains a coma
Line 65	commas—dates, Rule 4
Line 65	comma—conjunction, Rule 3
Lines 66, 67	commas—dates, Rule 4

PATIENT: Edward Carson   ADMITTED: 5/17/–
CHART #:   DISCHARGED: 5/30/–

HISTORY OF PRESENT ILLNESS:
This baby was 37 weeks of gestation and was born at Manning
Hospital on May 16, –, at 18:40. He was born by C-section for
nonreassuring fetal tones. Also, the non-stress test was non-reactive,
and there was a history of a previous C-section. The mother was a
24-year-old gravida 5, para 0-2-3, hepatitis B surface antigen negative,
A positive, **VDRL** nonreactive, rubella immune, and
group B streptococci negative. Pregnancy was complicated by
polyhydramnios, gestational diabetes, fetal tachycardia, and by
physical profile 2/8. C-section was done on May 16, –. The baby
was born at 18:40. Then, the baby after being delivered was
transferred to the Manning Hospital newborn nursery. Before
10 p.m. the baby was noted to be **tachypneic** and grunting. He was
placed on nasal CPAP and continued requiring oxygen the next day.
His ABGs in the morning showed a pH of 7.37, PCO_2 44, PO_2 132,
bicarb 26, and base excess of 0.6. At that time, assessment by the
pediatrician was at 37 weeks of gestation **LGA** born to diabetic
mother with probable **TTN**. The chest x-ray showed ground-glass
appearance. Blood cultures were done. Then on May 17,—, the
baby developed an episode of **tachycardia**. An **EKG** was performed
by Dr. Edward Weeks who diagnosed the baby with **supraventricular**
tachycardia. The baby was transferred without any problems
to St. Malachy's Hospital on May 17, –, and was admitted around
l o'clock to this unit.

REVIEW OF SYSTEMS

RESPIRATORY STATUS:
The baby required nasal CPAP. By the next day, the baby was off
the nasal CPAP and continued with a nasal cannula. He remained
on the nasal cannula until day of life #10. He was with nasal cannula
and oxygen until day #11 when he was placed for another 48 hours
on regular nasal cannula with no oxygen at 1 liter per minute. Then
on the last three days he was off oxygen saturating well with no
problems. Followup chest x-ray shows no infiltrate and normal
cardiac silhouette. The baby is breathing comfortably now without
any distress. Around day of life #5, the baby developed frequent
episodes of central apnea and clinically showed to be less active.
A complete sepsis workup done at this time showed to be negative.
Three days prior to discharge, the baby was started on caffeine after
a four-channel study showed frequent episodes of periodic breathing
and central apnea with desaturations.

43   CARDIOVASCULAR:
44   On admission, this baby was treated initially with **adenosine** which
45   did not have any effect on the supraventricular tachycardia and
46   then on propanolol which converted the baby to normal sinus
47   rhythm. Echocardiogram demonstrated a mild right atrium and
48   right ventricle **dilatation** and an adequate **myocardium** performance.
49   Another finding was prolonged **Q-T** of 452. After the periods of
50   supraventricular tachycardia, the next day a few other episodes were
51   noted which were **transient**. The baby gradually showed to be back
52   again to a normal sinus rhythm. The baby's cardiovascular status
53   continued improving. The Q-T continued decreasing in time. By
54   the time of discharge, according to cardiology, the EKG was less
55   than 400.

56   FEEDING AND NUTRITION:
57   The baby was initially **n.p.o.** After he was clinically stable, feedings
58   were introduced, and the baby tolerated his feedings well.

59   GASTROINTESTINAL:
60   No organomegaly. Blood sugar remained stable.

61   HEMATOLOGICALLY:
62   The baby never had any major complication. His last **H&H** was
63   15/43.8 with a normal platelet count and a normal white blood
64   cell count. His electrolytes were stable also. His sodium on
65   May 17, –, was 139 and on May 18, –, 143. His potassium was 4,
66   and a heel stick on May 18, –, showed 5.8. Bicarb was 24 on
67   May 17, –, and 25 on May 18, –.

68   INFECTIOUS DISEASE:
69   Complete sepsis workup did not show any gross abnormalities.
70   Viral cultures done on the rectal and nasopharyngeal looking
71   for **Enterovirus** and coxsackie virus are pending at this point.

72   MEDICATIONS:
73   The baby is on propanolol 2 mg **q8h** and caffeine 18 mg per day.

74   SOCIAL:
75   We had discussed the findings and the fact that the baby is improving
76   with the family. The prolonged Q-T and the risk of **SIDS** were dis-
77   cussed also.

78   **PLAN:**
79   The baby is going home on a home apnea monitor for the next 9
80   months. He is going to be followed by the pediatric cardiologist
81   and at the apnea clinic in 6 to 8 weeks.

82   _____
83   Mary Benoff, MD

84   MB/vs

85   d: 5/30/–   Word Count 768
86   t: 5/30/–   DSNEOEC.3

Caucasian		Pertaining to the white race.
hypoglycemia		A deficiency of blood sugar.
hypothyroid		Marked by insufficient thyroid secretion.
dysthymia		A chronically depressed mood that is present more than 50% of the time for at least 2 years in adults or 1 year for children or adolescents.
prognosis		Prediction of the cause and end of disease and estimated chances of recovery.

PUNCTUATION REFERENCES

Line 6	hyphens—compound modifier, Rule 1
Line 11	comma—conjunction, Rule 3
Line 13	commas—series, Rule 1
Line 18	apostrophe—singular possessive, Rule 1
Line 22	comma—introductory, Rule 7
Lines 27 and 28	quotation marks—exact words of speaker
Line 31	comma—conjunction, Rule 3
Line 33	comma—appositive, Rule 7
Line 33	semicolon—two independent clauses containing commas
Line 34	comma—appositive, Rule 7
Line 36	comma—appositive, Rule 7
Line 37	semicolon—two independent clauses, one containing a comma
Line 44	comma—introductory, Rule 7
Line 57	comma—conjunction, Rule 3
Line 63	semicolon—two independent clauses, one containing a comma
Line 63	comma—introductory, Rule 7
Line 72	comma—introductory, Rule 7
Line 73	hyphen—compound word, Rule 5
Line 78	hyphens—compound word, Rule 5
Line 80	apostrophe—contraction for "she is"
Line 80	comma—conjunction, Rule 3
Line 84	dash—words set off for emphasis
Line 87	comma—conjunction, Rule 3
Line 90	comma—conjunction, Rule 3
Line 92	comma—conjunction, Rule 3

1 NAME: Catherine DeLeo   MEDICAL RECORD NO.: 42-67-44
2 DATE: 5/31/–

3 OPINION AND RECOMMENDATIONS:

4 HISTORY:
5 The patient was seen on 5/31/– between the hours of 17:00 and
6 18:25. The patient is a 33-year-old **Caucasian** woman who was
7 admitted to Manning Hospital on 5/28/– because of difficulty in
8 controlling her care for diabetes. She has a history of having an
9 eating disorder with some element of depression. History is given
10 by the patient stating that she has been depressed for the past
11 three years, and for the past four months she has been taking
12 300 mg per day of Effexor. She describes herself as being very
13 irritable, crying a lot, and being generally unhappy. She denies
14 any sleep disturbance except that she gets up frequently to
15 urinate because she drinks much water. Appetite is impaired
16 by her eating disorder.

17 She states that she first began noting emotional problems after
18 witnessing her mother's sudden death from asthma when the
19 patient was age 13. She was then raised by her grandmother.
20 She graduated from Carlton High School. She attended Bryant
21 Tech College and graduated in 19– with a degree in marketing.
22 Afterwards, she worked in marketing for Delta Air Lines. She was
23 working prior to the recent onset of problems.

24 FAMILY HISTORY:
25 She has one brother age 35. She resides with her father in Coral
26 Heights. She describes him as never having been around when
27 she needed him in the past and states that he is "very nice but
28 a bit limited."

29 She has been treated for depression with Zoloft and Paxil prior
30 to using Effexor. She has had some psychiatric treatment in the
31 past. While she was in high school she saw a therapist, but she
32 feared that there was no direction or guidance from this person.
33 In college she saw Dr. John Allen, a psychologist; and after college
34 she saw Dr. Lillian Larkin, a psychologist in Bryant Park. She saw
35 her for two years. She was started on Zoloft and subsequently
36 Paxil by Dr. Marks and then began seeing Dr. Gordon Ling,
37 another psychologist; but she feels that she was not really
38 changing.

39 She has had an eating disorder since adolescence and has
40 fluctuated in weight. She stated that her present weight was
41 130 pounds with a height of 69 inches but that six years ago
42 she weighed 200 and several months ago weighed only 113.

PHYSICAL EXAMINATION:

On mental examination, she seemed very critical of herself. She thought of herself as being fat even though she did not appear to be so. Her weight was considered adequate at this time though she still eats what she wants to eat and when she wants to eat it. She very often limits herself and drinks much water to satisfy her hunger. She is diabetic and was diagnosed as such two years ago and is insulin dependent. She was well oriented. She denied hallucinations. Delusions were not elicited. She was able to recall six digits forward and five in reverse on digit span testing. She spoke quite eloquently and coherently and showed what I considered an appropriate emotional reaction to what she was speaking about though she was quite preoccupied that she was not happy in her present state of life. She was still living at home, and she had no relationship with any man and no prospects of marriage. She stated that boyfriends had been a problem with her family because they did not approve of people she would date. She stated that she has much difficulty controlling insulin coverage and described having had four episodes of **hypoglycemia** which she was able to abort by eating fruit. There is definitely a problem in eating; and to address this, she was referred from here after her last admission to an eating disorder treatment center in Philadelphia. It was there that she was started on Effexor. She had also been diagnosed **hypothyroid** and is taking Synthroid 50 mg per day. It is also noted that she takes Propranolol 1 mg twice a day and Allegra 180 mg per day.

IMPRESSION:

Dysthymia and an eating disorder mixed.

It is advised that the dose of Effexor be increased to 350 mg per day. If she has no benefit from this within a week, Desipramine at 25 mg twice a day should be started with an eventual build-up to 75 mg per day in doses of 25 mg each. She should be under the care of a psychiatrist who would be able to both prescribe medication and do psychotherapy with insight therapy and investigative therapy of her emotions in the past and her relationship with her family leading to present self-image. This self-image needs much improvement. She has little faith in herself. She does not think she's attractive though she is, and she considers herself to be obese which she is definitely not. She denies any suicidal

82 ideas. I do not believe she requires hospital care for the psychiatric
83 condition though she will require close following for the care of the
84 diabetes—another reason to be under the care of a psychiatrist who
85 could assist in monitoring this rather than the psychologist or lay
86 therapist. There may well be a problem with health coverage in this
87 regard, but it is essential that the person treating her be a physician
88 to control medication for her depression. She will have to be
89 referred to or find someone on her own who would be willing to
90 work with her HMO in this regard, or she would have to pay for
91 the treatment herself.

92 **Prognosis** is guarded for the depression, but it is quite possible
93 that she can be helped to achieve more of what she wants in life.

94 Thank you for the privilege of this consultation.

95 _____
96 Harry A. Peters, MD

97 HAP/rf

98 d: 5/31/—   Word Count 840
99 t: 5/31/—   CONPSYCD.1

defibrillator	An electric device that produces defibrillation of the heart.
echocardiogram	The graphic record produced by echocardiography (a noninvasive diagnostic method that uses ultrasound to visualize internal cardiac structure).
transesophageal	Through the esophagus.
subjugated	Submissive and without control.
dysrhythmia	Abnormal, disordered, or disturbed rhythm.
habituating	Habit-forming.

PUNCTUATION REFERENCES

Line 4	hyphens—compound modifier, Rule 1
Line 12	comma—introductory, Rule 7
Line 14	comma—conjunction, Rule 3
Line 15	comma—introductory, Rule 7
Line 18	comma—conjunction, Rule 3
Line 21	commas—parenthetical, Rule 10
Line 24	comma—introductory, Rule 7
Line 26	comma—conjunction, Rule 3
Line 26	hyphen—for clarification
Line 28	comma—introductory, Rule 7
Lines 34 and 35	commas—contrasting statement, Rule 12
Line 38	hyphen—for clarification
Line 42	comma—conjunction, Rule 3
Line 44	commas—series, Rule 1
Lines 46, 47	commas—series, Rule 1
Line 49	comma—conjunction, Rule 3
Line 59	comma—introductory, Rule 7
Line 59	semicolon—one independent clause contains a comma in a compound sentence.
Line 60	comma—introductory, Rule 7
Lines 60, 61	commas—series, Rule 1
Line 65	hyphen—compound word, Rule 4
Line 69	hyphen—compound modifier, Rule 1

Line 73	hyphen—for clarification
Line 74	comma—conjunction, Rule 3
Line 75	hyphen—compound modifier, Rule 1
Line 77	apostrophe—singular possessive, Rule 1
Line 78	hyphen—compound modifier, Rule 1
Line 79	comma—conjunction, Rule 3
Line 83	commas—parenthetical, Rule 10
Line 88	comma—conjunction, Rule 3
Line 89	hyphen—written fraction, Rule 2
Line 90	commas—parenthetical, Rule 10

NAME: Joan McDonald   MEDICAL RECORD NO.: 65-13-74
DATE: 9/7/

OPINION AND RECOMMENDATIONS:
This 30-year-old Caucasian female was seen in her room at the
request of Dr. Lang in psychiatric consultation because of anxiety.
She has had to have a planned implantation of a **defibrillator**
and is quite anxious about this.

HISTORY:
History was taken primarily from the patient. She stated that she
was well until the third week of July. She had had a previous
echocardiogram in June of this year which was said to be normal.
In July she began noticing fatigue. By the second week of August,
she noted some migraine headaches while flying as a flight
attendant. These were treated, and they subsided. By the third
week of August, she felt an increase in fatigue while vacationing
in Nantucket and had difficulty pursuing her usual activities. On
8/31/– she was noted to have a rapid heart rate of 170 beats per
minute when checked by her physician, and she was advised
admission here.

Electrophysiological studies were performed. On Friday of last
week, according to her, she went into ventricular fibrillation during
an electrophysiological study and was immediately shocked while
awake to bring her out of this. While partially sedated under the
influence of Versed and morphine, she went into ventricular
tachycardia again and was shocked for the second time. These
events left her quite stressed, and for two days she kept re-living
the incidents and became very anxious in the process. On the
following Monday, she tolerated a cardiac biopsy procedure. She
stated that she had had a previous **transesophageal** echocardiogram
performed and that she recalled sobbing violently throughout the
procedure even though she was under sedation. She was told that
she fought off the people who were performing it. She has little
recollection of this. She is told now that she requires a defibrillator
and is very fearful, not of the operation, but of the testing of the
defibrillator. She fears that it might possibly go off again and that
she would be **subjugated** again to the stress of electrostimulation.
She is quite fearful of this. She has had no nightmare concerning
the episode but does have considerable anxiety in re-living the
experience and in thinking about what may happen in the future.

Her past psychiatric history shows evidence of much trauma in her
childhood and adolescence as a result of family problems. Her father
had affairs, and this led to considerable problems with the mother.

43   The mother would confide in the patient and sought solace from
44   her. This left the patient tense, anxious, and distressed. Many of
45   these problems have been resolved. She saw various therapists
46   within the past ten to twelve years in Los Angeles, Miami, New
47   York, and Connecticut and has had considerable help from them.
48   She is now able to relate to her parents better. They divorced
49   when she was 16 in 19–, and she still sees and is close to both
50   sides of the family. Both parents have remarried.

51   Personal history was that she was born in Maine but lived most of
52   her life in Connecticut. She graduated from high school there. She
53   was a fairly good student. She attended college for two years at
54   Jones University in Massachusetts. She worked for a bank for two
55   years before joining the airlines as a stewardess or flight attendant.
56   She has been working for Globe Airlines since 19–. She had an
57   accident falling off a horse prior to beginning her job and fractured
58   her pelvis. Her job went well until the Globe Airlines strike by
59   employees in 19–. After this, management became more strict, and
60   the job was less pleasant to her. However, she does enjoy the salary,
61   the benefits, and the frequent times off. She returned to school at
62   Eastern Connecticut State in 19– and obtained her degree. She is
63   also interested in working now in a radio station where she had
64   worked part-time in 19—. She would eventually like to do this
65   full-time. She states that there could be a problem working there
66   because there are demagnetizers used which have a rather strong
67   magnetic field and might be a problem with the defibrillator.
68   She has agreed to discuss this with her cardiologist.

69   Mental status examination shows a well-oriented woman. She
70   denies hallucinations. Delusions were not elicited. She describes
71   the anxiety as mentioned above. She has not had nightmares
72   concerning the defibrillating experiences with the electric shocks
73   but has re-lived it many times especially for the two days after
74   it happened. This is decreasing, but there is continued anxiety.

75   This woman has a long-standing history of psychoneurotic
76   personality problems. There is also a family history of cardiac
77   problems on the mother's side.

78   The present diagnosis is acute post-traumatic stress disorder.
79   Prognosis is good, but there is a residual fear of repeating the shock

80 experience. She realizes she may have to live through this. It is
81 advised that any procedures where shock will be used should be
82 tested under as much anesthesia as possible to avoid a repetition
83 of electroshock with her being awake. It is understood, of course,
84 that this would not be possible if the defibrillator is activated by
85 cardiac **dysrhythmia** while she is awake. She hopes her medication
86 will be sufficient to prevent this.

87 Thank you for the courtesy of this consultation. I have
88 discontinued Xanax with its **habituating** potential, and I
89 have replaced it with clonazepam (Klonopin) 0.5 mg one-half
90 tablet twice a day, only if needed, for severe anxiety. The patient
91 will be followed in psychiatric support and therapy while she
92 is here.

93 _____
94 Barton Mandelberg, MD

95 BM/kl

96 d: 9/7/—   Word Count 840
97 t: 9/7/—   CONPSYJM.2

Consultation Reports

OVERVIEW

In this section the student will be transcribing consultation reports specific to the endocrine, female reproductive, gastrointestinal, genitourinary, and lymphatic body systems.

Terminology previews are provided for each report. Punctuation references illustrating uses of the comma, hyphen, semicolon, and colon are provided in four reports.

CONSULTATION REPORTS

Physicians request consultation reports from other physician specialists to assist in a comprehensive diagnosis of the patient's illness or disease. Consultations may be restricted to one body system or may be a thorough examination of the total patient.

Consultation reports may be in correspondence format or follow the same general pattern as the history and physical examination report. The consultation reports that follow are in correspondence format, using a modified block style, blocked paragraphs, mixed punctuation, and a subject line with the patient's name following the salutation.

Use of Macros

It is recommended that the student prepare a macro on a word processor to contain the subject line, "Patient:," and another macro for the complimentary closing, "Sincerely yours,". The first macro can be named and retrieved with "Alt p"; the second macro can be named and retrieved with "Alt s." (Consult your instructional manual for macro preparation, as needed.)

Multiple Page Headings

When the letter/report exceeds one page, key the patient's name, and page number, and date, beginning on the first line of each succeeding page. For example,

Mary Smithson

Page 2

February 14, 20–

Saving and Coding Transcripts

The student should name and save each transcribed report with the code provided at the end of each report.

INSTRUCTIONAL OBJECTIVES

In this chapter, the student will:

1. Transcribe consultation reports of varying lengths in letter format.
2. Learn terminology relative to the endocrine, female reproductive, gastrointestinal, genitourinary, and lymphatic body systems.
3. Reinforce understanding of the use of comma (introductory, series, conjunction, day/year, city/state, title/person's name, parenthetical, complimentary closing), hyphen (compound modifier), semicolon (independent clauses without a comma and conjunction, independent clauses when the second clause begins with a transitional expression), and colon (business letters).

REMINDERS: Preview highlighted medical terms and punctuation references in the report.
Listen to the tape to become familiar with it.
Transcribe the report inserting punctuation "cues."
Print out a hard copy.
Check carefully your transcribed report word by word to the text transcript.

THE TRANSCRIPT IN THE TEXT IS CHECKED <u>ONLY AFTER</u> YOU HAVE COMPLETED YOUR TRANSCRIPTION.

Record the number of lines transcribed and the number of minutes needed to complete the report.
Make corrections; submit the corrected transcript to your instructor.

CONSULTATION REPORTS INDEX

	Patient Name	Code Name	Word Count
END	WILLIAM SARKAR	CONENDWS.1*	169
	JENNIFER ADAMS	CONENDJA.2	292
FEM	HEATHER FLEMMING	CONFEMHF.1	174
	JANET HOLSLEY	CONFEMJH.2	207
	ELIZABETH SINGER	CONFEMES.3	210
	CYNTHIA FOSTER	CONFEMCF.4	206
	DANIELLE TANTA	CONFEMDT.5	234
GAS	SEAN A. ROGERS	CONGASSR.1	129
	SAMANTHA BROWNE	CONGASSB.2	175
	TAYLOR GREEN	CONGASTG.3	185
	GENE COMPUTO	CONGASGC.4*	221
	JERMAINE SHARMEN	CONGASJS.5*	274
GEN	ANTHONY CANNETTA	CONGENAC.1	103
	PETER DISPLARD	CONGENPD.2	108
	MORTON ANEAR	CONGENMA.3	236
LYM	VIRGINIA TREVORS	CONLYMVT.1	239
	MIRA SOMLYO	CONLYMMS.2*	300

*Punctuation References

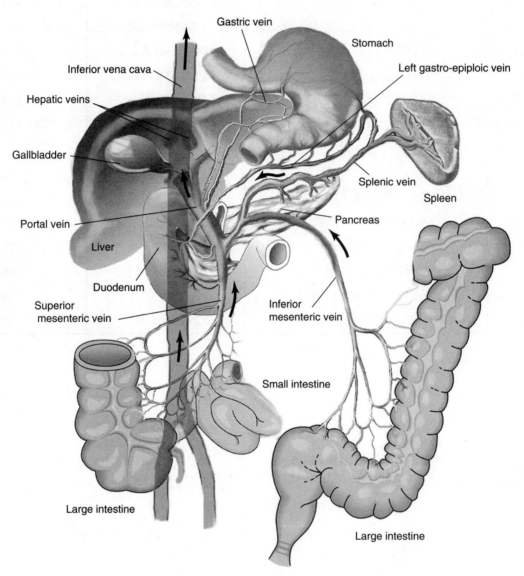

Gastric vein

Stomach

Inferior vena cava

Left gastro-epiploic vein

Hepatic veins

Gallbladder

Splenic vein

Spleen

Portal vein

Pancreas

Liver

Duodenum

Superior
mesenteric vein

Inferior
mesenteric vein

Small intestine

Large intestine

Large intestine

Portal circulation

CONENDWS.1	William Sarkar	Terminology Preview
sacroiliac		Relating to the sacrum and the ilium.
metastatic		Relating to the shifting or spreading of a disease, or its local manifestations, from one part of the body to another.
lymphadenopathy		Any disease process affecting a lymph node or lymph nodes.
periceliac		Relating to around the abdominal cavity.
portacaval		Concerning the portal vein and the inferior vena cava.
periaortic		Surrounding or adjacent to the aorta.
retroperitoneum		External or posterior to the peritoneum (tissue that lines the abdominal cavity).

PUNCTUATION REFERENCES

Line 1	comma—day and year, Rule 4
Line 2	comma—titles that follow a person's name, Rule 7
Line 4	comma—city and state, Rule 5
Lines 5, 6, 8	colon—business letters, Rule 4
Line 14	comma—day and year, Rule 4
Lines 19, 20	commas—series, Rule 1
Line 22	colon—business letters, Rule 4
Line 26	comma—complimentary closing, Rule 9
Line 27	comma—titles that follow a person's name, Rule 7

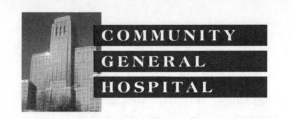

10 Main Street

Yourtown, NY, 10000

(000) 000-0000

May 9, 20—

Alison J. Kelly, MD
4578 East 92 Street
Brooklyn, NY 11235

Dear Dr. Kelly:

Patient: William Sarkar

The following radiologic procedure was performed on your patient: CT ABDOMEN.

Multiple CT images were obtained from the xiphoid through the superior aspect of the **sacroiliac** joints following the oral and intravenous administration of contrast.

A comparison is made with the previous study dated April 12, 20—. The current scan reveals that the **metastatic** lesion is identified in the left adrenal gland measuring approximately 4.4 cm. In addition, there is extensive new bulky **lymphadenopathy** in the **periceliac** and **portacaval** regions as well as in the **periaortic** area of the **retroperitoneum**. The liver, spleen, pancreas, and kidneys remain normal in appearance.

IMPRESSION: Marked progression of metastatic disease involving the adrenal glands bilaterally and retroperitoneal and upper abdominal lymph nodes.

Thank you for referring this patient for consultation.

Sincerely yours,

Marcus Q. Turner, MD

MQT/urs

d: 5/8/—
t: 5/9/—

Word Count 169
CONENDWS.1

CT	Computed tomography.
metastatic	Relating to the shifting or spreading of a disease, or its local manifestations, from one part of the body to another.
benign	Denoting the mild character of an illness or the nonmalignant character of a neoplasm.
adenoma	An ordinarily benign neoplasm of epithelial tissue in which the tumor cells form glands or glandlike structures in the stroma (the framework, usually of connective tissue, of an organ, gland, or other structure); usually well circumscribed, tending to compress rather than infiltrate or invade adjacent tissue.

1   December 12, 20–

2   Daniel Moses, MD
3   1357 Sixth Avenue
4   New York, NY 10123

5   Dear Dr. Moses:

6   Patient: Jennifer Adams

7   The following radiologic procedure was performed on
8   your patient: **CT** ABDOMEN/PELVIS.

9   A CT scan of the abdomen and pelvis was performed
10   following the oral and intravenous administration
11   of contrast.

12   No abnormalities are seen within the liver, spleen, or
13   pancreas. There is a 1.5 cm in diameter mass in the
14   region of the right adrenal gland. From this
15   particular study, it is uncertain whether this actually
16   represents an adrenal mass, or a mass in the liver, or
17   at the upper pole of the kidney.

18   We cannot make a definite distinction because a routing
19   scan of the abdomen was performed, and comparatively
20   large sections were obtained through this portion of
21   the abdomen making definition as to exactly where this
22   mass resides unclear.

23   If it is in the adrenal, it could represent a
24   **metastatic** focus of disease in view of the clinical
25   history, or it may represent an incidental **benign**
26   **adenoma**. A definite statement as to this
27   differentiation cannot be made, and further evaluation
28   is indicated.

29   The remaining portions of this scan including the
30   abdomen and pelvis are entirely normal. There is no
31   evidence of metastatic disease or other abnormalities
32   seen.

Jennifer Adams
Page 2
December 12, 20—

33 IMPRESSION: A 1.5 cm mass in the region of the right
34 adrenal gland which needs further evaluation as outlined in
35 the report. This could represent a metastatic process although
36 the possibility of an incidental benign adenoma might also
37 give this picture. Possibly, a more detailed CT scan would be
38 necessary to help make the differentiation.

39 Thank you for referring this patient for consultation.

40   Sincerely yours,

41   Sheng Jeung, MD

42 SJ/urs

43 d: 12/11/—
44 t: 12/12/—   Word Count 292
45 📼   CONENDJA.2

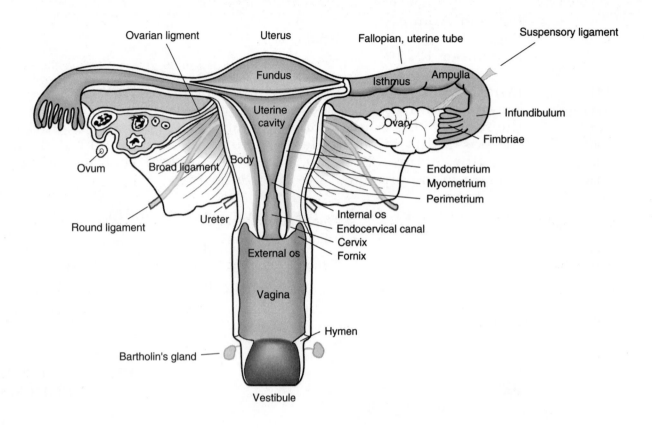

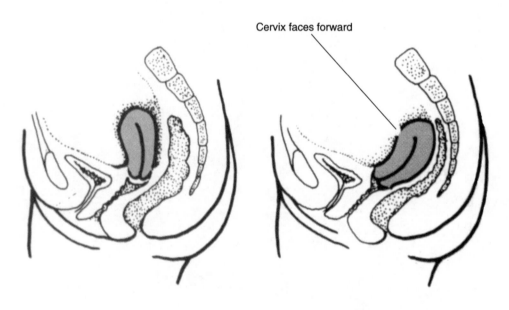

Retroversion

Marked Retroversion

Cervix faces forward

Female reproductive system

SONO	Sonogram.
endovaginally	Within the vagina, the genital canal in the female, extending from the uterus to the vulva.
unilocular	Having but one compartment or cavity, as in a fat cell.
adnexal	Relating to parts accessory to the main organ or structure (appendage).
cyst	An abnormal sac containing gas, fluid, or a semisolid material with a membranous lining.
ovarian follicle	One of the spheroidal cell aggregations in the ovary containing an ovum.
retroverted	Denoting a turning backward, as of the uterus.
endometrial stripe	A streak, line, band, or stria relating to or composed of the mucus membrane comprising the inner layer of the uterine wall.

1   October 3, 20—

2   William T. Prescott, MD
3   1294 Millhouse Street
4   New York, NY 10012

5   Dear Dr. Prescott:

6   Patient: Heather Flemming

7   The following radiologic procedure was performed
8   on your patient: **SONO** PELVIS.

9   A real-time ultrasound examination of the pelvis was
10   performed **endovaginally**.

11   A **unilocular** right **adnexal cyst** remains unchanged in
12   comparison to prior ultrasound examinations and
13   measures approximately 4.3 cm in length × 4 cm in
14   anterior posterior dimension × 4.3 cm in transverse
15   dimension.

16   The right ovary measures approximately 3.4 × 2.3
17   × 2.7 cm. An **ovarian follicle** measuring approximately
18   2.1 × 1.6 × 1.7 cm is identified.

19   At least four follicles are identified within the left
20   ovary. These all measure less than 1 cm in **diameter**.
21   The uterus is **retroverted** in position. Normal
22   **endometrial stripe** is demonstrated.

23   IMPRESSION: A 2.1 × 1.6 × 1.7 cm right ovarian follicle.
24   A stable 4 cm right adnexal cyst.

25   Thank you for referring this patient for consultation.

26   Sincerely yours,

27   Maria Jethwani, MD

28   MJ/urs

29   d: 10/3/—
30   t: 10/3/—
31   ■⌣■

                                                    Word Count 174
                                                    CONFEMHF.1

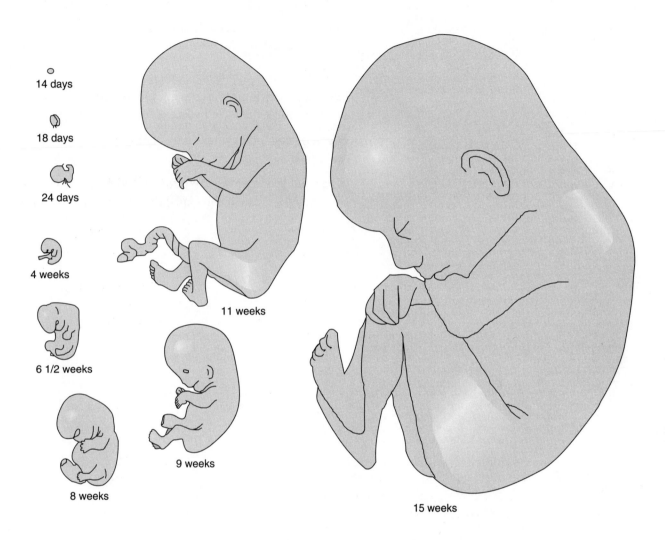

14 days

18 days

24 days

4 weeks

6 1/2 weeks

8 weeks

9 weeks

11 weeks

15 weeks

Changes in the body size of the embryo and fetus during development in the uterus (all figures natural size).

Embryonic/fetal development

intrauterine pregnancy	Gestation with the development of a fetus or fetuses within the uterus.
gestational	Pertaining to the length of time of development and growth from conception to birth.
amniocentesis	Transabdominal (through or across the abdomen or abdominal wall) aspiration of fluid from the amniotic sac.
gravid	Pregnant.
breech	Reversed position of fetus where fetal buttocks present rather than the head.
placenta	Organ of metabolic interchange between fetus and mother.
BPD	Biparietal (concerning the two parietal bones that form the roof and sides of the skull) diameter of fetal head.

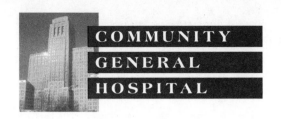

COMMUNITY
GENERAL
HOSPITAL

10 Main Street

Yourtown, NY, 10000

(000) 000-0000

1   September 28, 20—

2   Bridget T. Young, MD
3   294 Housing Avenue
4   New York, NY 10035

5   Dear Dr. Young:

6   Patient: Janet Holsley

7   The following radiologic procedure was performed on
8   your patient: SONO AMNIOCENTESIS.

9   DIAGNOSIS: 1. Single live **intrauterine pregnancy** of estimat-
10   ed **gestational** age 17.5 weeks +/− 10 days.

11   2. Successful ultrasound-guided
12   **amniocentesis** was performed.

13   COMMENTS: A real-time ultrasound examination of the
14   **gravid** uterus was performed. A single live intrauterine
15   pregnancy is present.

16   The fetus is in a **breech** lie. The **placenta** is
17   posterior, Grade 0. Amniotic fluid volume is within
18   normal limits for the estimated gestational age. **BPD**
19   40.7, head circumference 141, abdominal circumference 130,
20   femur length 26.4 correspond to an estimated
21   gestational age of 17.5 weeks +/− 10 days. Fetal
22   anatomic survey demonstrated lateral ventricles,
23   stomach, cord insertion, bladder, and spine to be
24   grossly normal in appearance. A four-chamber view of
25   the heart was obtained. The fetal heart motion and
26   fetal movements were observed pre- and post-amniocentesis.

27   A successful ultrasound-guided amniocentesis was
28   performed in a single pass by Dr. Bruce Young.

29   Approximately 20 cc of clear amniotic fluid
30   was withdrawn.

Janet Holsley
Page 2
September 28, 20—

31   Thank you for referring this patient for consultation.

32   Sincerely yours,

33   Lyla C. Kaplan, MD

34   LCK/urs

35   d: 9/27/—
36   t: 9/28/—   Word Count 207
37   CONFEMJH.2

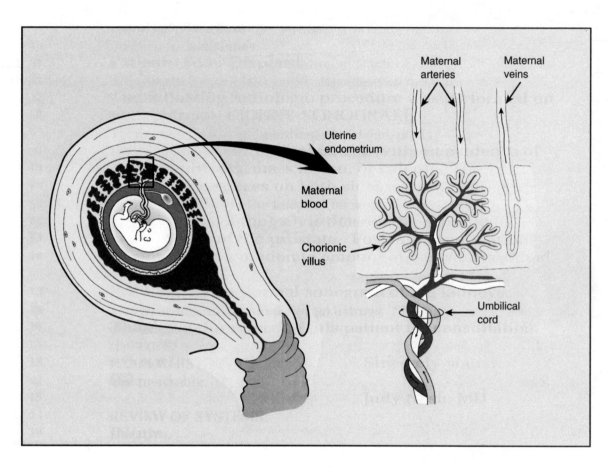

Fetal circulation

amniocentesis	Transabdominal aspiration of fluid from the amniotic sac.
intrauterine pregnancy	Gestation with the development of a fetus or fetuses within the uterus.
gestational	Relating to the length of time of development and growth from conception to birth.
lateral	Pertaining to the side.
fundal	Pertaining to the body of the uterus above the openings of the fallopian tubes.

August 12, 20–

Lois C. Kaplan, MD
494 Tenth Street
New York, NY 10007

Dear Dr. Kaplan:

Patient: Elizabeth Singer

The following is a radiologic procedure performed on your patient: SONO **AMNIOCENTESIS**

DIAGNOSIS: 1. Single live **intrauterine pregnancy** of estimated **gestational** age 17.5 to 18 weeks +/− 10 days.

2. Successful ultrasound guided amniocentesis was performed.

COMMENTS: A real-time ultrasound examination of the gravid uterus was performed. A single live intrauterine pregnancy is present.

The fetus is in a breech lie. The placenta is right **lateral** and **fundal** in location, grade 0. Amniotic fluid volume is within normal limits for the estimated gestational age. BPD 42, head circumference 145, abdominal circumference 121, and femur length 25.5 correspond to a composite estimated gestational age of 17.5 to 18 weeks +/− 10 days. Fetal anatomic survey demonstrated lateral ventricles, stomach, cord insertion, bladder, and spine to be grossly normal in appearance. A four-chamber view of the heart was obtained. Fetal heart motion and fetal movements were observed pre- and post-amniocentesis.
A successful ultrasound-guided amniocentesis was performed in a single pass by Dr. Kevin Lang. Approximately 20 cc of clear amniotic fluid was withdrawn.

Elizabeth Singer
Page 2
August 12, 20—

33   Thank you for referring this patient for consultation.

34   Sincerely yours,

35   Florence Coppland, MD

36   FC/urs

37   d: 8/12/—
38   t: 8/12/—   Word Count 210
39   ▣   CONFEMES.3

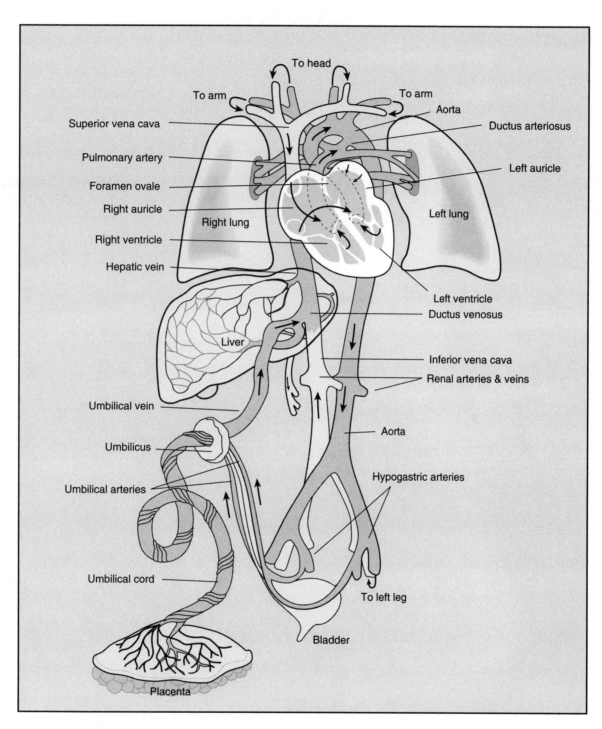

Maternal-fetal circulation

SONO	Sonogram.
amniocentesis	Transabdominal aspiration of fluid from the amniotic sac.
intrauterine pregnancy	Gestation with the development of a fetus or fetuses within the uterus.
gravid	Pregnant.
placenta	Organ of metabolic interchange between fetus and mother.
anteriorly	Refers to the ventral or abdominal side of the body.
posteriorly	Refers to the rear or caudal end of the body; opposite of anterior.

October 6, 20–

Nicholas Wolf, MD
650 Broadway
New York, NY 10007

Dear Dr. Wolf:

Patient: Cynthia Foster

The following radiologic procedure was performed on your patient: **SONO AMNIOCENTESIS**

DIAGNOSIS: 1. Single live **intrauterine pregnancy** of estimated gestational age 15 weeks +/– one week.

2. Amniocentesis has been rescheduled. A detailed fetal anatomic survey can be performed at that time.

COMMENTS: A real-time ultrasound examination of the **gravid** uterus was performed. A single live intrauterine pregnancy is present.

The fetus is in a variable lie. The **placenta** is left lateral and wraps **anteriorly** and **posteriorly**. The placenta is grade 0. Amniotic fluid volume is within normal limits for the estimated gestational age.

BPD 32, head circumference 114, abdominal circumference 93, and femur length 18.3 correspond to a composite estimated gestational age of 15 weeks +/– one week.

Fetal anatomic survey was limited at this time; however, lateral ventricles and stomach appeared grossly normal. Further anatomic detail regarding visualization of cord insertion, fetal urinary bladder, and spine can be obtained when the patient returns for amniocentesis. Fetal heart motion and fetal movements were observed.

Cynthia Foster
Page 2
October 6, 20—

31   Thank you for referring this patient for consultation.

32   Sincerely yours,

33   Bernard J. Churner, MD

34   BJC/urs

35   d: 10/5/—
36   t: 10/6/—   Word Count 206
37   CONFEMCF.4

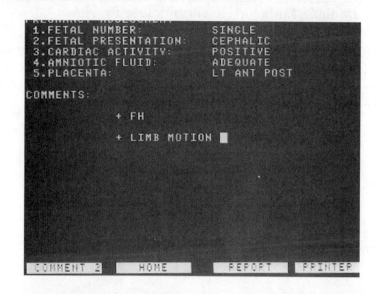

```
PREGNANCY ASSESSMENT
 1.FETAL NUMBER:          SINGLE
 2.FETAL PRESENTATION:    CEPHALIC
 3.CARDIAC ACTIVITY:      POSITIVE
 4.AMNIOTIC FLUID:        ADEQUATE
 5.PLACENTA:              LT ANT POST

COMMENTS:

        + FH

        + LIMB MOTION ■

 COMMENT 3      HOME          REPORT     PRINTER
```

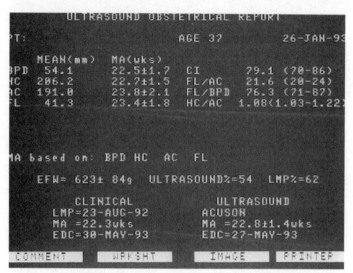

```
          ULTRASOUND OBSTETRICAL REPORT

PT:                     AGE 37          26-JAN-93

     MEAN(mm)   MA(wks)
BPD   54.1     22.5±1.7   CI       79.1 (70-86)
HC   206.2     22.7±1.5   FL/AC    21.6 (20-24)
AC   191.0     23.8±2.1   FL/BPD   76.3 (71-87)
FL    41.3     23.4±1.8   HC/AC    1.08(1.03-1.22)

MA based on: BPD HC  AC  FL

   EFW= 623± 84g   ULTRASOUND%=54   LMP%=62

       CLINICAL              ULTRASOUND
   LMP=23-AUG-92          ACUSON
   MA =22.3wks            MA =22.8±1.4wks
   EDC=30-MAY-93          EDC=27-MAY-93

 COMMENT       WRKSHT        IMAGE      PRINTER
```

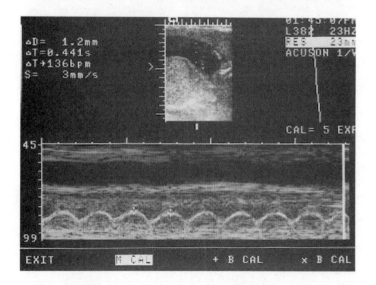

```
                              01:45:07PM
ΔD=   1.2mm                   L382   23HZ
ΔT=0.441s                     RES    23mm
ΔT→136bpm                     ACUSON 1/V
S=    3mm/s

                              CAL= 5 EXP
45

99
 EXIT         M CAL       + B CAL    x B CAL
```

Sonograms of fetal development (22nd week)

choroid plexus cysts	Closed sacs or pouches containing a network of blood or lymphatic vessels with dark brown vascular coat.

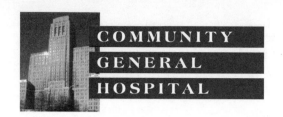

COMMUNITY GENERAL HOSPITAL

10 Main Street

Yourtown, NY, 10000

(000) 000-0000

1   September 26, 20—

2   Charles J. Poitner, MD
3   709 Pine Avenue
4   Brooklyn, NY 11245

5   Dear Dr. Poitner:

6   Patient: Danielle Tanta

7   The following radiologic procedure was performed on
8   your patient: SONO AMNIOCENTESIS

9   DIAGNOSIS: 1. Single live intrauterine pregnancy of
10   estimated gestational age of 17 weeks
11   +/— 10 days.

12   2. Bilateral **choroid plexus cysts**. Follow-up
13   ultrasound examination is recommended in
14   four weeks.

15   3. Successful ultrasound-guided
16   amniocentesis was performed.

17   COMMENTS: A real-time ultrasound examination of the
18   gravid uterus was performed. A single live intrauterine
19   pregnancy is present.

20   The fetus is in a breech lie. The placenta is posterior
21   and grade 0. Amniotic fluid volume is within normal
22   limits for the estimated gestational age.

23   BPD 38, head circumference 140, abdominal circumference
24   124, and femur length 25.6 correspond to a composite
25   estimated gestational age of 17 weeks +/— 10 days.

26   Fetal anatomic survey demonstrated lateral ventricles,
27   stomach, cord insertion, bladder, and spine to be grossly
28   normal in appearance. Bilateral choroid plexus cysts
29   measuring approximately 7 mm in diameter were present.
30   A four-chamber view of the heart was obtained. The fetal
31   heart motion and fetal movements were observed pre-
32   and post-amniocentesis.

Danielle Tanta
Page 2
September 26, 20—

33   A successful ultrasound guided amniocentesis was
34   performed in a single pass by Dr. Lara Thomas.
35   Approximately 20 cc of clear amniotic fluid
36   was withdrawn.

37   Thank you for referring this patient for consultation.

39   Sincerely yours,

41   Carolyn T. Smith, MD

43   CTS/urs

45   d: 9/26/—
46   t: 9/26/—   Word Count 234
47   ◼◼◼   CONFEMDT.5

barium enema	Administration of barium, a radiopaque (radiodense; impenetrable to the x-ray or other forms of radiation) medium for radiographic study of the lower intestinal tract.
fluoroscopic	Relating to or effected by means of fluoroscopy (examination of the tissues and deep structures of the body by x-ray, using the fluoroscope).
cecum	About 6 cm in depth, lying below the terminal ileum forming the first part of the large intestine.
ileocecal valve	Sphincter muscles that serve to close the ileum at the point where the small intestine opens into the ascending colon. It prevents food material from re-entering the small intestine.

MANNING MEDICAL CENTER
1 HOMETOWN, ANYWHERE, CA, 00001

1 June 30, 20—

2 Claudia T. Smith, MD
3 1230 West 34 Street
4 New York, NY 10163

5 Dear Dr. Smith:

6 Patient: Sean A. Rogers

7 The following radiologic procedure was performed on
8 your patient: **BARIUM ENEMA**.

9 A double contrast barium enema examination was
10 performed under **fluoroscopic** control using high-density
11 barium and air.

12 Barium flowed freely from rectum to **cecum** with
13 visualization of the **ileocecal valve**. A small amount
14 of retained fecal material was seen throughout the
15 colon, but no definite constant intrinsic or extrinsic
16 filling defects are seen.

17 The colon is normally distensible. No abnormalities
18 are noted.

19 IMPRESSION: Normal study.

20 Thank you for referring this patient for consultation.

21 Sincerely yours,

22 Edward J. Johnson, MD

23 EJJ/urs

24 d: 6/30/—
25 t: 6/30/—
26

Word Count 129
CONGASSR.1

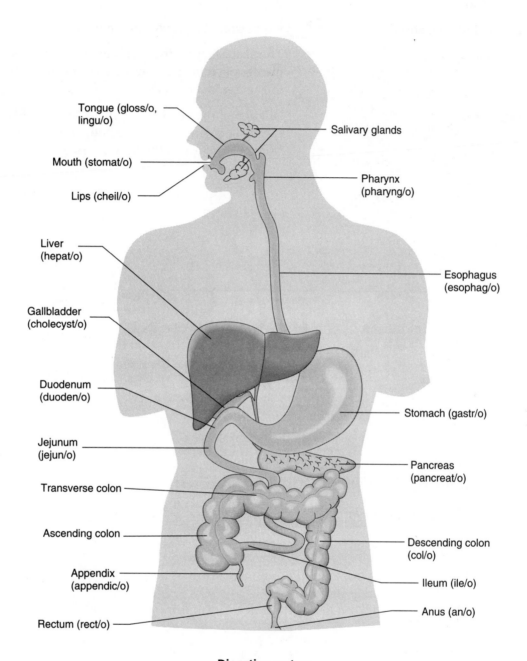

Digestive system

SONO	Sonogram.
cholecystectomy	Surgical removal of the gallbladder.
biliary dilatation	Increase of bile.
intrahepatic duct dilatation	Expansion of duct within the liver.
retroperitoneum	The space behind the peritoneum (the serous membrane reflected over the viscera and lining the abdominal cavity).
hydronephrosis	Dilation of the pelvis and calyces (any cuplike organs or cavities) of one or both kidneys resulting from obstruction to the flow of urine.

January 20, 20—

B. T. Henry, MD
4730 Redding Street
New York, NY 10007

Dear Dr. Henry:

Patient: Samantha Browne

The following radiologic procedure was performed on your patient: **SONO** LIVER

DIAGNOSIS: The patient is status post **cholecystectomy**. There is no evidence of **biliary dilatation**. There is a 6 cm left renal cyst.

COMMENTS: A real-time ultrasound examination of the abdomen was performed. The liver is normal in size and homogeneous in echo texture without evidence of focal mass or **intrahepatic duct dilatation**. The patient is status post cholecystectomy. The common bile duct is normal in caliber.

Evaluation of the **retroperitoneum** was limited, however, its size measures 12 cm in length. The left kidney measures 12.5 cm in length. There is a 6 cm midpole left renal cyst. The right kidney measures 10.5 cm in length. There are several small right renal cysts.

There is no **hydronephrosis**.

Thank you for referring this patient for consultation.

Sincerely yours,

Anne D. Higgins, MD

ADH/urs

d: 1/20/—
t: 1/20/—

Word Count 175
CONGASSB.2

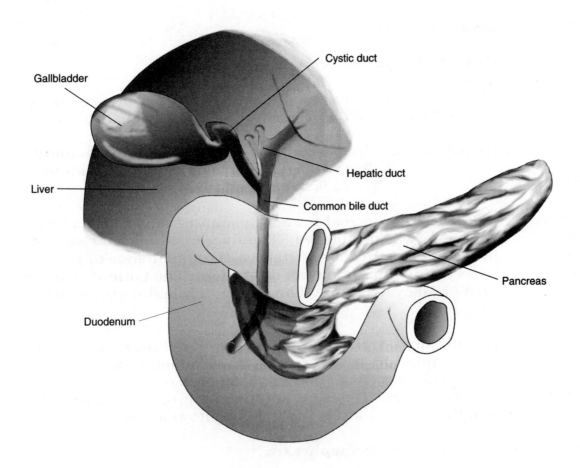

Gallbladder

Cystic duct

Liver

Hepatic duct

Common bile duct

Pancreas

Duodenum

Liver, gallbladder, and pancreas

focal	Starting point of a disease process.
intrahepatic duct dilatation	Expansion of duct within the liver.
renal calculus	Kidney stone.
anechoic	Sonolucent; echo-free; not containing internal interfaces that reflect high-frequency sound waves.
peripelvic cysts	Abnormal sacs containing gas, fluid, or semisolid material, with a membranous lining located around or about the pelvis.
hydronephrosis	Dilation of the pelvis and calyces of one or both kidneys resulting from obstruction to the flow of urine.
ascites	Accumulation of serous (producing or containing serum or a serumlike substance) fluid in the peritoneal cavity.

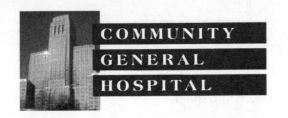

10 Main Street

Yourtown, NY, 10000

(000) 000-0000

1   November 5, 20—

2   F. John Outings, MD
3   545 First Street
4   New York, NY 10007

5   Dear Dr. Outings:

6   Patient: Taylor Green

7   The following radiologic procedure was performed on
8   your patient: SONO GALLBLADDER

9   DIAGNOSIS: 1. Fatty infiltration of the liver.

10   2. Right lower pole renal calculus.

11   COMMENTS: A real-time ultrasound examination of the
12   abdomen was performed. The liver is normal in size,
13   heterogeneous in echo texture, but increased in echogenicity.
14   The appearance is consistent with fatty infiltration of areas
15   with **focal** fatty spacing.

16   There is no evidence of **intrahepatic duct dilatation**.

17   The gallbladder is normal in size.

18   The right kidney measures 11.4 cm in length. There is
19   a small lower pole right **renal calculus**. The left
20   kidney measures 11 cm in length. Several **anechoic**
21   structures are identified within the central collecting
22   system of the left kidney. These do not appear to
23   communicate and are consistent in appearance with
24   several **peripelvic cysts**. There is no **hydronephrosis**.

25   There is no **ascites**.

Taylor Green
Page 2
November 5, 20—

26   Thank you for referring this patient for consultation.

27   Sincerely yours,

28   Jacquelyn Quentin, MD

29   JQ/urs

30   d: 11/5/—
31   t: 11/5/—   Word Count 185
32   CONGASTG.3

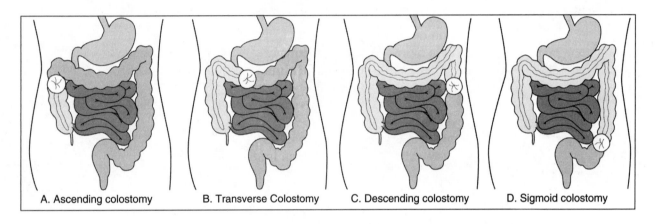

A. Ascending colostomy   B. Transverse Colostomy   C. Descending colostomy   D. Sigmoid colostomy

Colostomy sites

CONGASGC.4	Gene Computo	Terminology Preview
xiphoid		The lowest portion of the sternum; sword-shaped cartilaginous process supported by bone.
symphysis		The junction of the pubic bones on midline in front; the bony eminence under the pubic hair.
iliac artery		Artery related to the ileum (lower three-fifths of the small intestine from the jejunum to the ileocecal valve).
lymphadenopathy		Any disease process affecting a lymph node or lymph nodes.
retroperitoneum		The space behind the peritoneum.
abdominoperineal		Concerning the abdomen and perineal area (pelvic floor).
colostomy		Establishment of an artificial cutaneous (pertaining to the skin) opening into the colon.
prostate		A chestnut-shaped body, surrounding the beginning of the urethra in the male.
calcification		Deposition of lime or other insoluble calcium salts; a process in which tissue or noncellular material in the body becomes hardened.

PUNCTUATION REFERENCES

Line 1	comma—day and year, Rule 4
Line 2	comma—title following a person's name, Rule 7
Line 4	comma—city and state, Rule 5
Lines 5, 6, 8	colon—business letters, Rule 4
Lines 12, 13	commas—series, Rule 1
Line 15	semicolon—in place of comma and conjunction, Rule 1
Line 21	comma—conjunction, Rule 3
Line 34	comma—complimentary closing, Rule 9
Line 35	comma—title following a person's name, Rule 7

1   December 13, 20—

2   Lawrence J. Michaelson, MD
3   650 Broadway
4   New York, NY 10012

5   Dear Dr. Michaelson:

6   Patient: Gene Computo

7   The following radiologic procedure was performed on
8   your patient: CT ABDOMEN/PELVIS.

9   Multiple CT images were obtained from the **xiphoid**
10   through the **symphysis** following the oral and
11   intravenous administration of contrast.
12   The scans revealed the liver, spleen, pancreas,
13   adrenals, and kidneys to be normal in appearance.

14   A solitary 1 cm diameter lymph node is identified just
15   to the left of the left common **iliac artery**; this
16   solitary node is of uncertain significance.

17   No **lymphadenopathy** is seen in the **retroperitoneum** or
18   upper abdomen.

19   The patient is noted to be status post **abdominoperineal**
20   resection with transverse **colostomy**. A large amount
21   of fecal material is seen in the right colon, but there
22   is no definite radiographic evidence of bowel
23   obstruction.

24   Scans through the pelvis demonstrate multiple small
25   bowel loops in the rectal bed but no radiographic
26   evidence of recurrent disease.

27   The **prostate** is significantly enlarged and contains
28   multiple **calcifications**.

Gene Computo
Page 2
December 13, 20—

29   IMPRESSION: Status post abdominoperineal resection.
30   No definite evidence of recurrent disease. Solitary
31   1 cm retroperitoneal lymph node of uncertain
32   significance. There is prostatic enlargement.

33   Thank you for referring this patient for consultation.

34   Sincerely yours,

35   Amelia Graefenberg, MD

36   AG/urs

37   d: 12/13/—
38   t: 12/13/—   Word Count 221
39   ▰   CONGASGC.4

xiphoid	The lowest portion of the sternum; sword-shaped cartilaginous process supported by bone.
symphysis	The junction of the pubic bones on midline in front; the bony eminence under the pubic hair.
atrophic	Denoting atrophy (a wasting of tissues as from death and reabsorption of cells).
pseudocysts	Dilatations resembling cysts.
neoplasm	A new and abnormal formation of tissue, as a tumor or growth.
retroperitoneum	In back of the peritoneum.

PUNCTUATION REFERENCES

Line 12	commas—series, Rule 1
Line 14	hyphen—compound modifier, Rule 1
Line 18	comma—conjunction, Rule 3
Line 26	comma—introductory, Rule 7
Line 33	hyphen—compound modifier, Rule 1

October 18, 20—

James T. Feld, MD
6803 Fourth Avenue
New York, NY 10068

Dear Dr. Feld:

Patient: Jermaine Sharmen

The following radiologic procedure was performed on your patient: CT ABDOMEN/PELVIS.

Multiple CT images were obtained from the **xiphoid** through the **symphysis** following the oral and intravenous administration of contrast.

The scans revealed the liver, spleen, adrenals, and kidneys to be normal in appearance.

The pancreas is **atrophic**. There is a simple cystic-appearing lesion approximately 1.5 cm in diameter in relation to the tail of the pancreas. This most likely represents a simple pancreatic cyst or residual small **pseudocysts**, but the possibility of a small cystic **neoplasm** of the pancreatic tail cannot be excluded based on the CT appearance.

There is a cluster of slightly enlarged lymph nodes in the periaortic region just below the level of the crossing left renal vein. The largest node measures 1.5 cm in diameter.

Scans through the pelvis demonstrate no central masses. However, several slightly enlarged nodes are identified along both pelvic side walls measuring up to approximately 1.5 cm in diameter.

IMPRESSION: 1. Multiple slightly enlarged lymph nodes in the **retroperitoneum** and along both pelvic side walls.

Jermaine Sharmen
Page 2
October 18, 20—

32 IMPRESSION (continued): 2. Approximately 1.5 cm simple
33 cystic-appearing lesion in the tail of the pancreas. This most
34 likely represents a residual pseudocyst or simple pancreatic
35 cyst although the less likely possibility of a small cystic
36 pancreatic neoplasm cannot be entirely excluded.
37 Follow-up CT would be helpful for further evaluation
38 of this lesion.

39 Thank you for referring this patient for consultation.

40   Sincerely yours,

41   Everett Coopers, MD

42 EC/urs

43 d: 11/26/—
44 t: 11/27/—   Word Count 274
45   CONGASJS.5

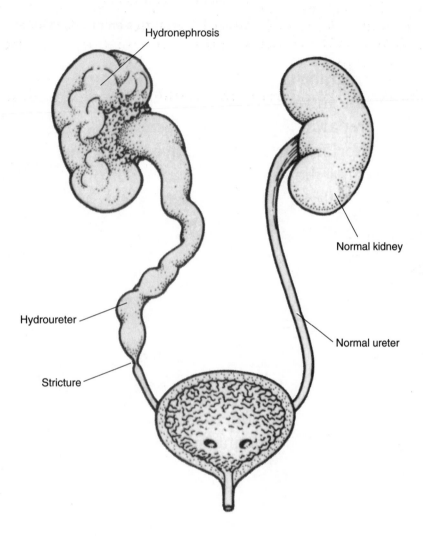

Urinary system pathology

hydronephrosis	Condition wherein there is a large, fluctuating, soft mass in the region of the kidney, appearing and disappearing as retained urine passes into the ureters and bladder (urine is collected in the renal pelvis due to obstructed outflow).
calculi	Commonly called stones.
perinephric	Located or occurring around the kidney.

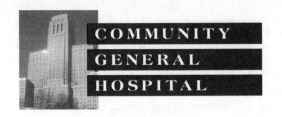

COMMUNITY

GENERAL

HOSPITAL

10 Main Street

Yourtown, NY, 10000

(000) 000-0000

1   April 7, 20—

2   Herbert B. Herring, MD

3   1209 Vine Avenue

4   Brooklyn, NY 11289

5   Dear Dr. Herring:

6   Patient: Anthony Cannetta

7   The following radiologic procedure was performed on

8   your patient: SONO KIDNEYS

9   DIAGNOSIS: Normal renal ultrasound.

10   COMMENTS: A real-time ultrasound examination of the

11   kidneys was performed.

12   The kidneys are normal in size measuring approximately

13   11 to 11.5 cm in length. There is no evidence of

14   **hydronephrosis, calculi,** or renal mass. There are no

15   **perinephric** fluid collections.

16   Thank you for referring this patient for consultation.

17   Sincerely yours,

18   Carlton P. Jones, MD

19   CPJ/urs

20   d: 4/7/—

21   t: 4/7/—   Word Count 103

22   📼   CONGENAC.1

hydronephrosis	Condition wherein there is a large, fluctuating, soft mass in the region of the kidney, appearing and disappearing as retained urine passes into the ureters and bladder (urine is collected in the renal pelvis due to obstructed outflow).
calculi	Stones, usually composed of salts of inorganic or organic acids, or of other material such as cholesterol.
perinephric spaces	Spaces surrounding the kidney in whole or part.
prostate	A chestnut-shaped body, surrounding the beginning of the urethra in the male.

MANNING MEDICAL CENTER
1 HOMETOWN, ANYWHERE, CA, 00001

1   March 21, 20–

2   Lorraine T. Stevens, MD
3   652 Broadway
4   New York, NY 10634

5   Dear Dr. Stevens:

6   Patient: Peter Displard

7   The following radiologic procedure was performed on
8   your patient: KIDNEY SONOGRAM.

9   Both kidneys are normal in size without evidence of
10   **hydronephrosis**, mass lesion, or **calculi**. The
11   **perinephric spaces** on both sides are unremarkable.

12   Examination of the pelvis demonstrates minimal
13   enlargement of the **prostate**. Postvoid examination
14   demonstrates a moderate amount of postvoid residual.

15   IMPRESSION: Normal sonogram of the kidneys.

16   Thank you for referring this patient for consultation.

17   Sincerely yours,

18   Judy Nash, MD

19   JN/urs

20   d: 3/21/–
21   t: 3/21/–   Word Count 108
22   ▆▆   CONGENPD.2

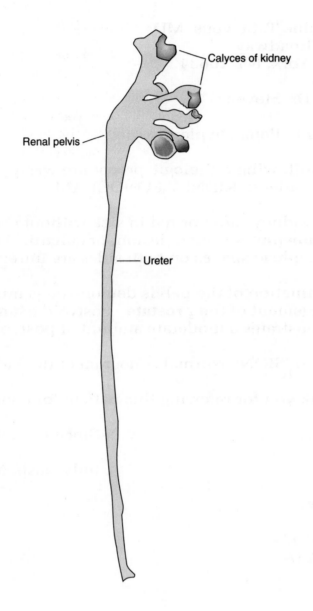

Calyces of kidney

Renal pelvis

Ureter

Kidney structures

contrast	A comparison in which differences are demonstrated or enhanced.
urogram	The roentgenographic record obtained by urography (roentgenography of any part—kidneys, ureters, or bladder—of the urinary tract).
calyces	Plural of calyx—any cuplike organ or cavity.
chronic	Of long duration; denoting a disease of slow progress and long continuance.
pyelonephritis	Inflammation of the renal parenchyma (the essential parts of an organ that are concerned with its function), calyces, and pelvis, particularly due to local bacterial infection.
reflux nephropathy	Condition wherein there is a backward flow of urine to the kidney.
adenopathy	Swelling or morbid enlargement of the lymph nodes.

June 4, 20—

Bernard J. Clarke, MD
43 West 23 Street
New York, NY 10012

Dear Dr. Clarke:

Patient: Morton Anear

The following radiologic consultation was performed on your patient: CT ABDOMEN.

A CT scan of the abdomen was performed following the oral administration of **contrast**.

The patient did not receive intravenous contrast because he had had an intravenous **urogram** six hours earlier. Contrast material was still seen within the collecting system at the time of the examination. Because of this, however, we are unable to say whether there are any stones within the left collecting system because of the contrast material that was still present. There is marked scarring of the left kidney which is also small in size. The scarring appears to be associated with **calyces** which would indicate that this represents **chronic pyelonephritis** or possibly chronic **reflux nephropathy**. The possibility of some underlying stone disease cannot be excluded. There are no other abnormal findings noted in the CT scan of the abdomen. The right kidney is normal in appearance. The other organs and structures are essentially unremarkable. There is no evidence of **adenopathy**.

IMPRESSION: Shrunken, scarred left kidney probably secondary to chronic pyelonephritis or reflux nephropathy.

No other definite abnormality is seen.

Morton Anear
Page 2
June 4, 20—

32   Thank you for referring this patient for consultation.

33   Sincerely yours,

34   Norma A. Klein, MD

35   NAK/urs

36   d: 6/4—
37   t: 6/4/—   Word Count 236
38   🎙   CONGENMA.3

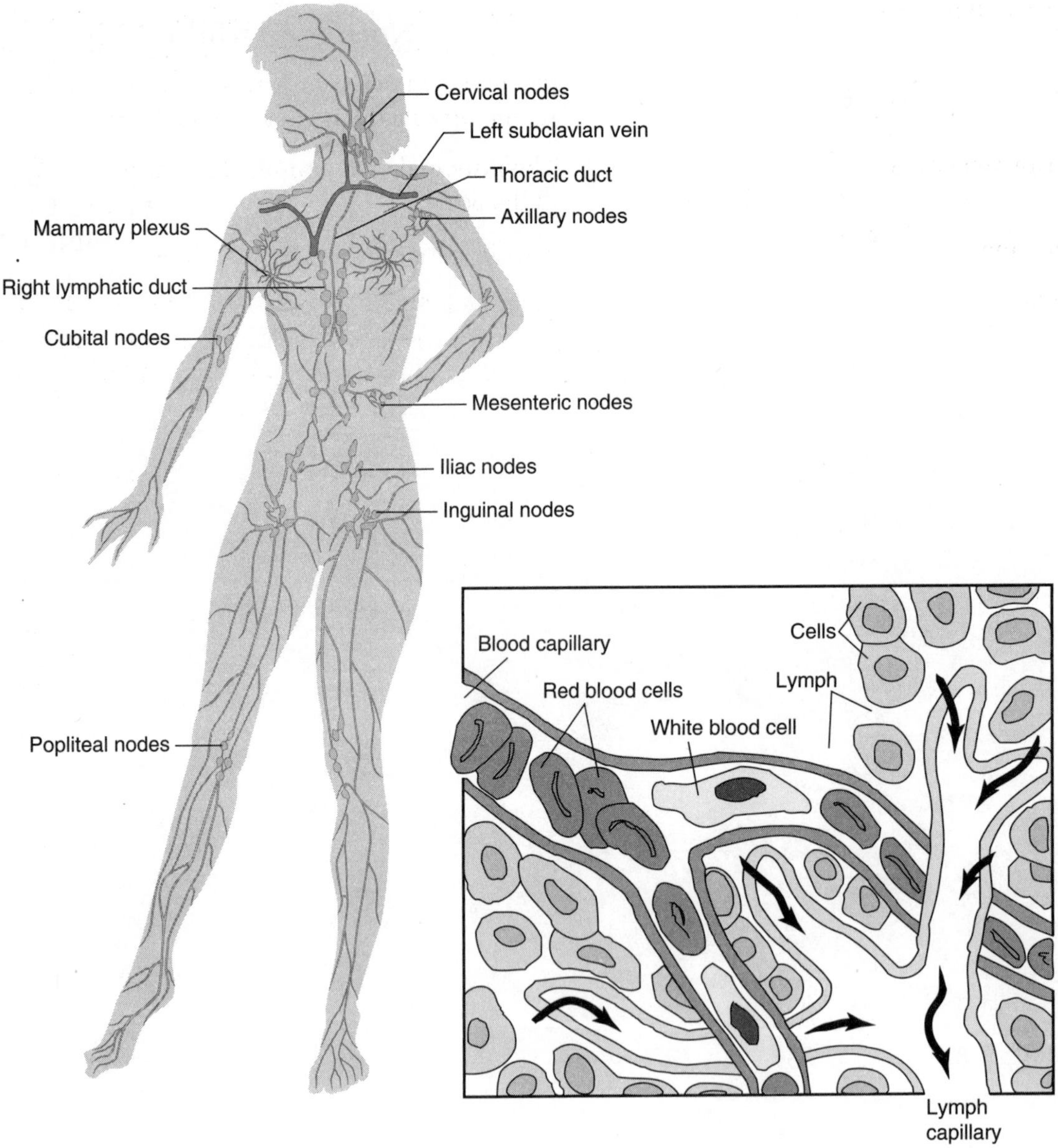
Cervical nodes
Left subclavian vein
Thoracic duct
Axillary nodes
Mammary plexus
Right lymphatic duct
Cubital nodes
Mesenteric nodes
Iliac nodes
Inguinal nodes
Popliteal nodes
Blood capillary
Cells
Lymph
Red blood cells
White blood cell
Lymph capillary

Lymphatic circulation

xiphoid	The lowest portion of the sternum; sword-shaped cartilaginous process supported by bone.
symphysis	The junction of the pubic bones on midline in front; the bony eminence under the pubic hair.
periaortic	Around the aorta.
pericecal lymphadenopathy	A disease process affecting a lymph node or lymph nodes in the area surrounding the cecum (about 6 cm in depth), lying below the terminal ileum forming the first part of the large intestine.
inferior vena cava	The principal vein draining the lower portion of the body.
duodenum	The first division of the small intestine.
fibrotic	Pertaining to or characterized by fibrosis (formation of fibrous tissue as a reparative or reactive process, as opposed to formation of fibrous tissue as a normal constituent of an organ or tissue).

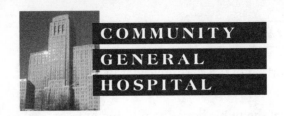

COMMUNITY

GENERAL

HOSPITAL

10 Main Street

Yourtown, NY, 10000

(000) 000-0000

1   July 23, 20–

2   Angela M. Clarke, MD
3   650 Broadway
4   New York, NY 10012

5   Dear Dr. Clarke:

6   Patient: Virginia J. Trevors

7   The following radiologic procedure was performed on
8   your patient: CT ABDOMEN/PELVIS.

9   Multiple CT images were obtained from the **xiphoid**
10   through the **symphysis** following oral and intravenous
11   administration of contrast.

12   A comparison is made with previous study dated June 15, 20–.
13   The current scan reveals **periaortic** and **pericecal**
14   **lymphadenopathy.**

15   The largest lymph node mass, to the left of the aorta,
16   now measures 3 × 2 cm. It had previously measured
17   4 × 2 cm.

18   There is a lymph node posterior to the **inferior vena**
19   **cava** at the level of the right renal vein. This had
20   previously measured 1 cm and now measures 1.5 cm.
21   An enlarged lymph node is also seen between the
22   inferior vena cava and third portion of the **duodenum;**
23   this had previously measured 1.4 cm and now measures
24   2.2 cm.

25   No new lymphadenopathy is seen. **Fibrotic** changes are
26   again noted in the small bowel mesentery. The liver,
27   spleen, pancreas, and adrenals remain normal
28   in appearance.

29   Bilateral renal cysts are again identified.

30   Scans through the pelvis are unremarkable.

Virginia J. Trevors
Page 2
July 23, 20—

31 IMPRESSION: Retroperitoneal lymphadenopathy. When
32 compared with the previous scan of June 15, some of these
33 lymph node masses have progressed in size, while others
34 have regressed.

35 Thank you for referring this patient for consultation.

36   Sincerely yours,

37   Valerie Kelly, MD

38 VK/urs

39 d: 7/21/—
40 t: 7/23/—   Word Count 239
41   CONLYMVT.1

xiphoid	The lowest portion of the sternum; sword-shaped cartilaginous process supported by bone.
symphysis	The junction of the pubic bones on midline in front; the bony eminence under the pubic hair.
adrenals	A triangular-shaped body covering the superior surface of each kidney (adrenal glands).
lymphadenopathy	Any disease process affecting a lymph node or lymph nodes.
mesentery	The fan-shaped fold of peritoneum encircling the greater part of the small intestine and attaching it to the posterior abdominal wall.
peristaltic contraction	Pertaining to the movement of the intestine or other tubular structure, characterized by waves of alternate circular contraction and relaxation of the tube by which the contents are propelled onward.
gastric leiomyoma	A benign neoplasm (a new and abnormal formation of tissue, as a tumor or growth) derived from smooth muscle relating to the stomach.
etiology	The science and study of the causes of disease and their mode of operation; pathogenesis.

PUNCTUATION REFERENCES

Line 16	hyphen—compound modifier, Rule 1
Line 19	hyphen—compound modifier, Rule 1
Line 21	semicolon—independent clauses when the second clause begins with a transitional expression, Rule 2
Line 21	comma—introductory, Rule 7
Line 23	commas—series, Rule 1
Line 34	comma—introductory clause, Rule 7

MANNING MEDICAL CENTER
1 HOMETOWN, ANYWHERE, CA, 00001

1   February 14, 20–

2   Henrietta Jameston, MD
3   6403 Second Avenue
4   Suite 6K
5   New York, NY 10012

6   Dear Dr. Jameston:

7   Patient: Mira Somlyo

8   The following radiologic procedure was performed on
9   your patient: CT ABDOMEN/PELVIS.

10   Multiple CT images were obtained from the **xiphoid**
11   through the **symphysis** following oral and intravenous
12   administration of contrast.

13   A report of a previous CT scan performed on June 19, 20– is
14   available although the scan itself is not available
15   for comparison.

16   The current scans reveal a low-density lesion
17   approximately 8 mm diameter in the medial segment of
18   the left lobe of the liver. An even smaller (less than
19   5 mm) low-density lesion is seen in the lateral segment
20   of the left lobe of the liver. These lesions are too
21   small for accurate CT density measurements; therefore,
22   their radiologic significance is not clear.

23   The spleen, pancreas, **adrenals**, and kidneys are normal
24   in appearance. No **lymphadenopathy** is identified in the
25   small bowel **mesentery**. Scans through the pelvis
26   demonstrate no central masses or side wall
27   lymphadenopathy.

28   There is bilateral inguinal lymphadenopathy. The
29   largest node measures 1.5 cm in diameter which is
30   smaller than the previously reported 3 cm.

Mira Somlyo
Page 2
February 14, 20–

31 There is an area of soft tissue prominence along the
32 greater curvature of the gastric body, measuring
33 approximately 2 cm in size. Although this may
34 represent a **peristaltic contraction**, the possibility of
35 a small **gastric leiomyoma** cannot be excluded.

36 IMPRESSION: 1. Bilateral inguinal lymphadenopathy
37 which appears smaller than the previous description
38 on June 19, 20–.

39 2. Two very small hepatic lesions of uncertain **etiology**
40 and significance.

41 3. An area of soft tissue prominence on the greater
42 curvature of the stomach whose appearance suggests
43 a small gastric leiomyoma.

44 Thank you for referring this patient for consultation.

45   Sincerely,

46   Herbert C. Clemens, MD

47 HCC/urs

48 d: 2/14/–
49 t: 2/14/–   Word Count 300
50 📼   CONLYMMS.2

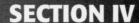

History and Physical Examination Reports

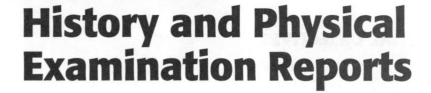

OVERVIEW

In this section the student will be transcribing history and physical examination reports specific to the cardiovascular, gastrointestinal, genitourinary, integumentary, and musculoskeletal body systems.

Terminology previews are provided for each report. Punctuation references illustrating uses of the comma, hyphen, semicolon, apostrophe, and dash are provided in three reports.

HISTORY AND PHYSICAL EXAMINATION REPORTS

History and physical examination reports are prepared on all hospitalized patients and outpatients in need of extensive evaluation.

Format Differences

There are several sections common to this type of report, but variations will occur depending upon the format preferences of the individual hospital. Most hospitals utilize preprinted forms containing sections for patient name, identification number, date, and other related data. These sections should be completed with the appropriate information.

While there are differences in the format of the history and physical examination report, all reports, at minimum, will have a section for the patient's history, physical examination, and/or impression, provisional diagnosis, and recommendation. The reports for transcription in this text illustrate some of these differences.

Use of a Macro

It is recommended that the student prepare a macro on a word processor to contain the heading, HISTORY AND PHYSICAL EXAMINATION, and the side headings for PATIENT: and CHART #:. The macro can be named and retrieved with "Alt h." (Consult your instructional manual for macro preparation, as needed.)

Multiple Page Headings

When the report exceeds one page, follow formatting style used by the hospital or key a heading to include the patient's name, chart number, and page number beginning on the first line of each succeeding page. For example,

Maude Kaufman

#987 654

Page 2

Saving and Coding Transcripts

The student should name and save each transcribed report with the code provided at the end of each report.

INSTRUCTIONAL OBJECTIVES

In this chapter, the student will:

1. Transcribe history and physical examination reports of varying lengths.
2. Learn terminology relative to the cardiovascular, gastrointestinal, genitourinary, integumentary, and musculoskeletal body systems.
3. Reinforce understanding of the use of comma (series, conjunction, two modifiers of same noun, parenthetical, and introductory), hyphen (compound modifier), semicolon (two independent clauses without a conjunction, two independent clauses with one or more clauses containing a comma), and dash (to give more emphasis to words).

REMINDERS: Preview highlighted medical terms and punctuation references in the report.
Listen to the tape to become familiar with it.
Transcribe the report inserting punctuation "cues."
Print out a hard copy.
Check carefully your transcribed report word by word to the text transcript.

THE TRANSCRIPT IN THE TEXT IS CHECKED <u>ONLY AFTER</u> YOU HAVE COMPLETED YOUR TRANSCRIPTION.

Record the number of lines transcribed and the number of minutes needed to complete the report.
Make corrections; submit the corrected transcript to your instructor.

HISTORY AND PHYSICAL EXAMINATION REPORTS INDEX

	Patient Name	Code Name	Word Count
CAR	RAJA HASHIMI	HPECARRH.1*	456
	LORI ASHLEY	HPECARLA.2	547
	JANICE OTTS	HPECARJO.3	565
GAS	LYLE LOCALI	HPEGASLL.1	187
	SYLVIA DOS SANTOS	HPEGASSD.2*	230
	SOFIA MARINE	HPEGASSM.3	395
	BELLA STANFORD	HPEGASBS.4*	437
	JAMES KIRKLAND	HPEGASJK.5	582
GEN	GORDON MAYERSON	HPEGENGM.1	197
	LEONARD NOBER	HPEGENLN.2	291
INT	ANN QUICKENS	HPEINTAQ.1	304
MUS	GLORIA WARD	HPEMUSGW.1	291
	JANE BROST	HPEMUSJB.2	364

*Punctuation References

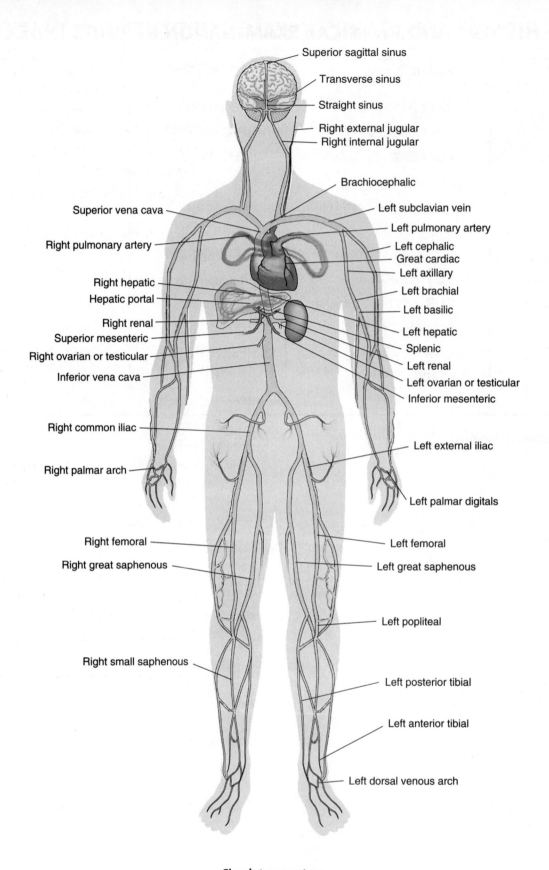

Superior sagittal sinus

Transverse sinus

Straight sinus

Right external jugular
Right internal jugular

Brachiocephalic

Superior vena cava

Left subclavian vein

Right pulmonary artery

Left pulmonary artery

Left cephalic
Great cardiac
Left axillary

Right hepatic
Hepatic portal

Left brachial

Left basilic

Right renal
Superior mesenteric
Right ovarian or testicular
Inferior vena cava

Left hepatic
Splenic
Left renal
Left ovarian or testicular
Inferior mesenteric

Right common iliac

Left external iliac

Right palmar arch

Left palmar digitals

Right femoral

Left femoral

Right great saphenous

Left great saphenous

Left popliteal

Right small saphenous

Left posterior tibial

Left anterior tibial

Left dorsal venous arch

Circulatory system

substernal	Below the sternum, or breastbone.
arteriosclerotic	Pertaining to a thickening and loss of elasticity of the arterial walls.
sick sinus syndrome	A complex cardiac arrhythmia (irregular heartbeat).
angina	Severe pain and constriction about the heart, usually radiating to the left shoulder and down the left arm.
myocardial infarction	Occlusion of one or more of the coronary arteries (heart attack).
herniorrhaphy (singular)	Surgical procedure for hernia repair.
claudication	Lameness, limping.
dyspnea	Difficult, labored breathing.
GI	Gastrointestinal.
GU	Genitourinary.
bruits	Sound, murmur heard in auscultation (process of listening for sounds within the body, usually of the thoracic or abdominal viscera, in order to detect some abnormal condition).
aVF	Augmented voltage unipolar left foot lead (electrocardiography).
cardiomegaly	Hypertrophy (increase in size of heart resulting from hypertrophy of muscle tissue, but without increase in size of cavities) of the heart.
nifedipine	A calcium channel blocker used as a coronary vasodilator, causing relaxation of the blood vessels, in the treatment of angina pectoris (severe pain and constriction about the heart, usually radiating to the left shoulder and down the left arm. Caused by an insufficient supply of blood to heart).
angiogram	Radiograph of blood vessel.

PUNCTUATION REFERENCES

Line 3	hyphen—compound modifier, Rule 1
Line 4	comma—to separate two modifiers of same noun, Rule 2
Line 13	commas—series, Rule 1
Line 23	commas—series, Rule 1
Line 27	semicolon—two independent clauses without a conjunction, Rule 1
Lines 30, 31	commas—series, Rule 1
Line 35	comma—conjunction, Rule 3
Line 39	comma—conjunction, Rule 3
Line 48	comma—conjunction, Rule 3
Lines 52, 53	dash—to give more emphasis to words, Rule 1

1 PATIENT: Raja Hashimi
2 CHART #:

3 HISTORY: The patient is a 72-year-old male who was
4 admitted because of intermittent, moderately severe
5 chest pain starting from the **substernal** region
6 radiating to the back and to the left arm and
7 associated with a choking sensation. The pain lasted
8 from minutes to half an hour and was relieved by two
9 nitroglycerin tablets.

10 This condition has been going on for the last two
11 weeks. The patient has known **arteriosclerotic** heart
12 disease and since his discharge in July 20–, has been doing
13 reasonably well on Procardia, nitrates, Persantine,
14 and digoxin.

15 PAST HISTORY: The patient had a pacemaker implantation
16 for **sick sinus syndrome** four years ago. He has a
17 history of **angina** and **myocardial infarction**. He also
18 has essential hypertension.

19 His past surgical history includes an appendectomy and
20 bilateral **herniorrhaphies**. He has no allergies.

21 The patient still works as a projectionist in a movie
22 house. He does not smoke but drinks occasionally. He
23 denies any history of diabetes, liver, or kidney
24 disease. There is no evidence of **claudication**.
25 The patient has exertional and nonexertional angina.
26 There is **dyspnea** on exertion and fatigability. **GI** is
27 negative; **GU** is negative.

28 PHYSICAL EXAMINATION: The patient is out of distress
29 right now. He has been given two injections of
30 Demerol. Blood pressure is 120/68, ventricular rate is
31 72 per minute, and respiratory rate is 60 per minute.
32 Color is good. Skin is warm. Examination of the head
33 shows that right lenticular opacity is greater than the
34 left. Neck veins are flat. There are no **bruits**.
35 Carotids are brisk, and there is no evidence of thyroid
36 enlargement. The heart is regular with no S3 gallops.
37 There is a systolic ejection murmur at the base III/VI.
38 The lungs are clear. The abdomen showed surgical
39 scars. Extremities have no edema. Pulses are 2+, and
40 there is no calf tenderness.

41   IMPRESSION: Unstable angina secondary to coronary
42   artery disease with obstructive and mixed pattern spasm
43   on an affixed lesion. Status post pacemaker
44   implantation and degenerative joint disease with
45   cervical degenerative arthritis.

46   Review of the EKG shows nonspecific ST-T wave changes
47   in II, III, and **aVF** and in the anterolateral leads.
48   Chest x-ray showed **cardiomegaly**, and the enzymes
49   are pending.

50   RECOMMENDATIONS: The patient should be hospitalized in
51   the coronary care unit and monitored. The **nifedipine**
52   should be increased up to 60 mg—slowly. Continue
53   Persantine. Continue transderm nitro—increase to 10.
54   Monitor the blood level. Consider **angiogram** when he
55   is stabilized.

56

57   _____

           Anita Bennock, MD

58   AB/urs

59   d: 11/2/–
60   t: 11/2/–   Word Count 456
61   ▄▄   HPECARRH.1

transient ischemic attack	Temporary or passing symptoms typically due to diminished blood flow through the brain.
arteriosclerotic heart disease	Pertaining to a thickening and loss of elasticity of the walls of the arteries in the heart.
arrhythmia	Irregular heart action.
osteoarthritis	Degenerative joint disease.
chronic organic brain syndrome	A large group of acute and chronic mental disorders associated with brain damage or impaired cerebral function.
paroxysmal atrial fibrillation	A sudden, periodic attack or recurrence of disease symptoms with extremely rapid, incomplete contractions of the atria resulting in fine, rapid, irregular, and uncoordinated movements.
APCs	Atrial premature contractions.
lethargic	Sluggish.
turgor	Resiliency.
hyperactive carotid pulse	Excessive activity pertaining to right and left common carotid arteries.
bruit	Sound or murmur heard in auscultation.
atelectasis	Collapsed or airless state of lung.
organomegaly	Enlargement of visceral organs.
edema	Accumulation of excess fluid in a body part.
polymorphonucleosis	A condition in which leukocytes (white blood corpuscles that act as scavengers, helping to combat infection) have nuclei consisting of several lobes.
SMA-6	Sequential Multiple Analysis—six different serum tests.
BUN	Blood, urea, nitrogen (BUN is a blood test that measures the blood level of urea; in kidney disease, the BUN results will be elevated indicating the kidneys' inability to excrete urea properly).
creatinine	Lab tests for measurement of kidney function.
ST-T	ST segment and T-waves (found on electrocardiograms).
myocardial infarction	Obstruction of blood supply to myocardium (the middle layer of the walls of the heart, composed of cardiac muscle) usually from occlusion of one or more of two large coronary arteries and their branches—commonly called a "heart attack."
idiopathic	Disease without recognizable cause, of spontaneous origin.
n.p.o.	Nothing by mouth.

1   PATIENT: Lori Ashley
2   CHART #:

3   HISTORY: The patient is an 87-year-old female who
4   was admitted yesterday because of weakness and
5   unresponsiveness.

6   The patient had been admitted recently to the hospital
7   for a diagnosis of **transient ischemic attack,**
8   **arteriosclerotic heart disease** and cardiac **arrhythmia.**
9   In addition, the patient had degenerative
10   **osteoarthritis** and **chronic organic brain syndrome.** The
11   patient could not give any history according to the
12   nurse's aide at home. The aide stated that the patient
13   had been unable to eat and had become weak, especially
14   on the right side. The patient started to gag on
15   feeding, and she was brought to the hospital for
16   further management and evaluation.

17   PAST HISTORY: This patient has arteriosclerotic heart
18   disease and hypertension. There was no evidence of
19   diabetes. There was no surgical history. There were
20   no known allergies. The family history was noncontributory.

21   During the last admission, the patient was disoriented
22   and confused. The patient was diagnosed as having
23   **paroxysmal atrial fibrillation** and a transient ischemic
24   attack. Persantine and digoxin were administered for
25   the atrial fibrillation and Pronestyl was started to
26   suppress the **APCs.**

27   PHYSICAL EXAMINATION: The patient was not in acute
28   distress, but was **lethargic.** She was nonverbal but
29   responded to painful stimuli. There was obvious
30   weakness of both right and left extremities.
31   The mouth showed a positive gag reflex. The neck had
32   distended neck veins. Skin **turgor** was poor.

33   There was a **hyperactive carotid pulse.** There was no
34   **bruit.** The heart had an atrial regular rhythm,
35   occasional premature beats, and some periods of
36   irregularity. A systolic ejection murmur was heard.
37   The chest was clear with some **atelectasis** on the
38   left base.

39   Blood pressure was 130/74. Ventricular rates ranged
40   from 60 to 80 per minute. The respiratory rate was
41   about 18 per minute.

42   The abdomen was soft. There were positive bowel
43   sounds; there was no **organomegaly**. Extremities had
44   no **edema**.

45   LABORATORY: The available data in the chart showed a
46   WBC count of 14,000 with **polymorphonucleosis**. However,
47   this could be on the basis of infection, either a
48   genitourinary or lung infection. The **SMA-6** was within
49   normal limits except for the **BUN** which has increased to
50   76. **Creatinine** was 2. There were elevated alkaline
51   phosphatase and triglycerides.

52   The EKG showed periods of sinus rhythm with multiple
53   APCs, **ST-T** wave abnormalities, short runs of paroxysmal
54   atrial fibrillation, and short runs of supraventricular arrhythmia.
55   There was no evidence of any acute **myocardial infarction**.
56   There were nonspecific ST-T changes. When compared with a
57   previous tracing, there were more ST-T wave abnormalities which
58   could be due to ischemia and/or digitalis effect.

59   The chest x-ray will be reviewed.

60   IMPRESSION: Diffuse cerebral dysfunction which is
61   probably on a cerebral arteriosclerotic basis. Paroxysmal
62   atrial fibrillation secondary to arteriosclerotic heart
63   disease. Rule out **idiopathic** hypertrophic subaortic
64   stenosis.

65   RECOMMENDATIONS: The patient should be **n.p.o.** for
66   the time being, and a neurological consultation should
67   be made.

68   Urine cultures will be evaluated.

69   Intravenous fluids should be provided, and the patient
70   considered for nasogastric tube feeding at a later date.

71

72   Antonio Chavez, MD

73   AC/urs

74   d: 11/4/—
75   t: 11/4/—   Word Count 547
76   📼   HPECARLA.2

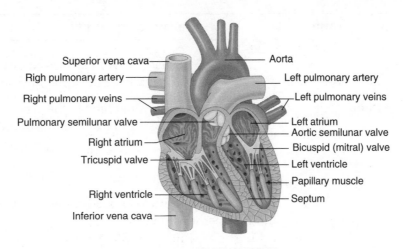

Superior vena cava — — Aorta
Righ pulmonary artery — — Left pulmonary artery
Right pulmonary veins — — Left pulmonary veins
Pulmonary semilunar valve — — Left atrium
— Aortic semilunar valve
Right atrium — — Bicuspid (mitral) valve
Tricuspid valve — — Left ventricle
— Papillary muscle
Right ventricle — — Septum
Inferior vena cava —

HEART ANATOMY

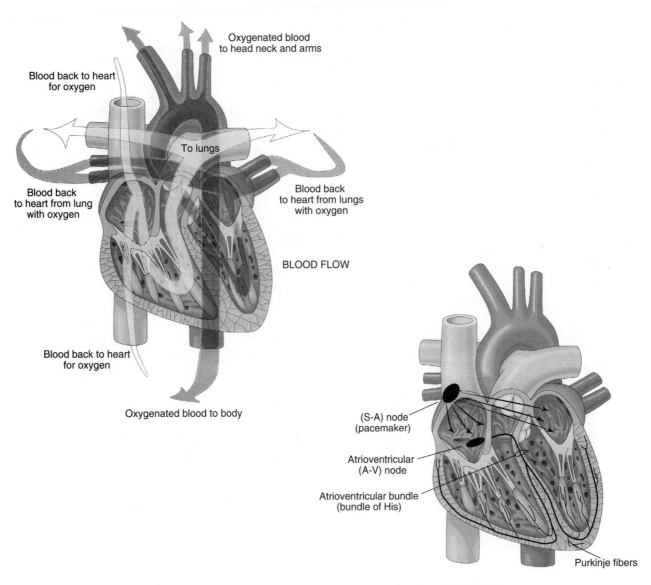

Oxygenated blood
to head neck and arms

Blood back to heart
for oxygen

To lungs

Blood back
to heart from lung
with oxygen

Blood back
to heart from lungs
with oxygen

BLOOD FLOW

Blood back to heart
for oxygen

Oxygenated blood to body

(S-A) node
(pacemaker)

Atrioventricular
(A-V) node

Atrioventricular bundle
(bundle of His)

Purkinje fibers

ELECTRICAL CONDUCTION

Heart anatomy; blood flow; electrical conduction

atrial fibrillation	Cardiac arrhythmia marked by rapid, irregular contractions of the atrial myocardium.
mitral regurgitation	Backflow of blood to the orifices of the heart due to imperfect closing of the mitral valve.
cardiomegaly	Hypertrophy of the heart.
dyspnea	Labored, difficult breathing.
orthopnea	Ability to breathe easily only in an upright position.
claudication	Lameness or limping.
hemoptysis	Coughing or spitting up of blood.
GI	Gastrointestinal.
GU	Genitourinary.
fundus	Base or bottom of an organ.
bruits	Sounds or murmurs heard in auscultation.
rales	Abnormal sound heard on auscultation.
holosystolic	Pertaining to entire systole.
hepatomegaly	Liver enlargement.
edema	Accumulation of excess fluid in a body part.
atelectatic	Pertaining to collapsed, airless state of lung.
PVCs	Premature ventricular contractions.
CBC	Complete blood cell count.
diuretics	Agents to increase urine secretion.
azotemia	Presence of nitrogen-containing compounds in the blood.

HISTORY AND PHYSICAL EXAMINATION

1   PATIENT: Janice Otts

2   CHART #:

3   HISTORY: This is one of several admissions for this

4   78-year-old female who has a known history of

5   congestive heart failure, **atrial fibrillation**, aortic

6   valve disease, and **mitral regurgitation.**

7   The patient had been admitted one week ago because of

8   episodes of increased shortness of breath and weakness.

9   At the time of her discharge, she was doing reasonably

10   well, controlled on digoxin and transderm nitro.

11   PAST HISTORY: The patient denies any history of

12   rheumatic fever. She has a history of hypertension,

13   arteriosclerotic heart disease with several episodes of

14   congestive heart failure, and atrial fibrillation with

15   **cardiomegaly**. There are no known allergies. Present

16   medication at this hospital consists of digoxin 125 mg.

17   Lasix was discontinued. The patient is also on

18   potassium supplementation.

19   REVIEW OF SYSTEMS: Cardiovascular: The patient

20   denies any chest pain, however, she has a history of

21   **dyspnea** on exertion. Last night, the patient had

22   paroxysmal nocturnal dyspnea. The patient has

23   two-pillow **orthopnea** and no evidence of **claudication**

24   or pain in the legs.

25   Respiratory: No chronic cough or **hemoptysis**.

26   **GI** is negative; **GU** is negative.

27   Musculoskeletal: The patient has low back pain.

28   Neurological is negative.

29   PHYSICAL EXAMINATION: The patient is alert,

30   cooperative, and not in acute distress. Blood pressure

31   is 140/76, ventricular rate is 78 per minute, and

32   respiratory rate is 26 per minute and irregular.

33   The patient is lying more comfortably at a 30 degree angle.

34   Examination of the head shows the **fundus** is benign.

35   The pupils are equal. There is no jaundice. Neck

36   veins show slight distention at 30.° There are no
37   **bruits**. There is a thyroid nodule anteriorly the size
38   of a quarter which is palpable and movable. The chest
39   shows clear to percussion but has minimal **rales**.

40   The heart shows irregularity at a rate of 78 per minute.
41   There is a **holosystolic** murmur at the apex going to the
42   axilla, and an asystolic ejection murmur at the base.
43   There is no diastolic murmur, and there is no gallop.
44   The abdomen is soft. There is no **hepatomegaly**.

45   Extremities show the pulses as 3+, and there is no
46   evidence of **edema** or calf tenderness.

47   LABORATORY STUDIES: Initial chest x-ray indicates
48   cardiomegaly and no acute infiltrate, congestion, or
49   effusion, but some **atelectatic** bands at the lower lung
50   fields on the lateral side.

51   The patient has atrial fibrillation with a moderately
52   rapid ventricular response, an old anteroseptal wall
53   myocardial infarction, a few **PVCs**, and nonspecific
54   ST-T wave changes. The SMA–6 and SMA–12 persistently
55   show BUN ranging from 44 to 51. CO_2 is slightly
56   elevated. At times, the potassium is 5.8 which is
57   high. **CBC** is within normal limits.

58   IMPRESSION: The patient has episodes of congestive
59   heart failure with left ventricular failure, paroxysmal
60   nocturnal dyspnea secondary to arteriosclerotic heart
61   disease and hypertensive cardiovascular disease, atrial
62   fibrillation with markedly rapid ventricular response,
63   mitral regurgitation secondary to mitral valve disease,
64   aortic systolic ejection murmur, and transient past
65   ischemic attacks.

66   RECOMMENDATION: The patient should continue her
67   digoxin 125 mg daily and preload reduction transderm
68   nitro. The patient should also continue on **diuretics**
69   in the form of Lasix and/or Zaroxolyn because the BUN
70   is on the basis of prerenal **azotemia** due to poor
71   cardiac output on pre-existing mild renal failure.

72   The patient should have fluid restriction of 1200 cc
73   per day and a 2-gram sodium diet.

74   _____
75   Herman J. Potts, MD

76   HJP/urs

77   d: 9/5/—
78   t: 9/5/—   Word Count 565
79   HPECARJO.3

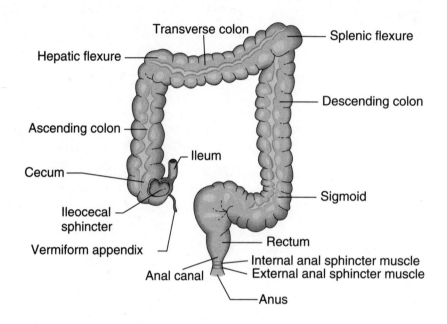

Large intestine

metastatic	Pertaining to the transfer of disease from one organ or part of the body to another not directly connected with it (spread is by the lymphatics or bloodstream).
carcinomatosis	The condition of widespread dissemination of cancer throughout the body.
umbilical hernia	Protrusion of abdominal contents through the abdominal wall at the umbilicus.
mucinous	Abnormal deposits of mucin (a glycoprotein found in mucus; it is present in saliva and bile and in salivary glands, in the skin, connective tissue, tendon, and cartilage) in the skin.
cystadenocarcinoma	Glandular malignancy that forms cysts as it grows.
prostatism	Any condition of the prostate gland that interferes with the flow of urine from the bladder.
transrectal	A surgical procedure through rectum.
5-FU	5-fluorouracil (chemotherapy, oncology, pharmacology).
leucovorin	Folinic acid (the calcium salt of folinic acid; it is used to antagonize the effect of Methotrexate on normal cells when Methotrexate is being used to treat malignancies).
HEENT	Head, eyes, ears, nose, throat.
conjunctivae	The delicate membranes lining the eyelids and covering the eyeballs.
sclerae	Whites of the eyes.
anicteric	Without jaundice.
fundi	The back portion of the interior of the eyeballs.
lymphadenopathy	Any disease process affecting the lymph nodes.
palpable	Perceptible to touch.
cyanosis	A bluish discoloration of the skin and mucous membranes due to reduced hemoglobin.
clubbing	Bulbous swelling of the terminal phalanges of the fingers and toes, giving them a "club" appearance.

HISTORY AND PHYSICAL EXAMINATION

1   PATIENT: Lyle Locali
2   CHART #:

3   ADMITTING DIAGNOSIS: **Metastatic** colon carcinoma
4   for chemotherapy.

5   HISTORY: The patient is a 54-year-old male who is
6   admitted for chemotherapy. The patient presented last
7   December with a metastatic **carcinomatosis** involving the
8   abdomen. The primary tumor was in the right colon. He
9   was diagnosed during a repair of an **umbilical hernia.**
10   The biopsy revealed a **mucinous cystadenocarcinoma.**

11   PAST HISTORY: The patient has **prostatism.** Multiple
12   **transrectal** biopsies of the prostate, however, did not
13   reveal any primary prostate cancer. The patient was
14   started on continuous infusion of **5-FU** and **leucovorin**
15   for his metastatic carcinomatosis. The patient is now
16   being admitted for his next cycle of chemotherapy.

17   PHYSICAL EXAMINATION: Blood pressure 120/80, pulse
18   80 and regular. **HEENT: Conjunctivae** pink, **sclerae**
19   **anicteric. Fundi**: Normal. ENT: Within normal
20   limits. No **lymphadenopathy**. Lungs: Normal.
21   Abdomen: Soft, nontender. Liver and spleen not
22   **palpable.** No abdominal masses noted. No vertebral
23   tenderness elicited. Extremities: No **cyanosis,**
24   **clubbing**, or edema.

25   IMPRESSION: Metastatic carcinoma of the colon.

26   _____
27   Stacy Peaks, MD

28   SP/urs

29   d: 6/28/—
30   t: 6/29/—   Word Count 187
31   ▣   HPEGASLL.1

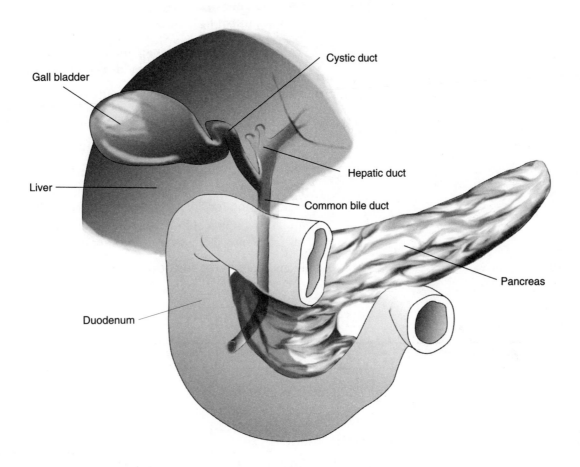

Gall bladder

Cystic duct

Liver

Hepatic duct

Common bile duct

Pancreas

Duodenum

Liver, gallbladder, and pancreas

gravida		A pregnant woman; called gravida 1 during the first pregnancy, gravida 2 during the second pregnancy, etc.
para		Used with numerals to designate the number of pregnancies that have resulted in the birth of viable offspring.
gallstones		Stonelike masses called calculi that form in the gallbladder.
jaundice		Yellowness of skin, sclerae, mucous membranes, and excretions due to gallbladder and liver disorder.
normocephalic		Pertaining to a normal, usual head.
atraumatic		Without trauma.
auscultation		Process of listening for sounds within the body.
guaiac negative		An alcoholic solution of guaiac is used to test for occult blood (a chemical test or microscopic examination for blood, especially in feces, that is not apparent on visual inspection) in feces. A negative test indicates there is no occult blood in feces.
cholecystectomy		Excision of the gallbladder.

PUNCTUATION REFERENCES

Line 4	hyphen—compound modifier, Rule 1
Line 4	commas—series, Rule 1
Line 7	comma—conjunction, Rule 3
Line 12	hyphen—compound modifier, Rule 1
Line 13	commas—series, Rule 1
Lines 27, 28	comma—parenthetical, Rule 10
Lines 28, 29	commas—series, Rule 1

1   PATIENT: Sylvia Dos Santos
2   CHART #:

3   HISTORY:
4   This is a 29-year-old, **gravida** 0, **para** 0, woman with a
5   history of right upper quadrant pain for a number of
6   months. The patient described the pain as severe and
7   sharp without radiation. The pain recurred, and the
8   patient went to her private medical doctor at which
9   point a sonogram was performed. The sonogram was
10   positive for **gallstones**.

11   The patient has not had pain for the last two months
12   while on a no-fat diet.

13   There is no history of **jaundice,** dark urine, or clay-
14   colored stool. There is no fever or chills.

15   PAST HISTORY:
16   Unremarkable.

17   ALLERGIES:
18   None.

19   SMOKING HISTORY:
20   The patient does not smoke or take drugs. She takes an
21   alcoholic drink occasionally.

22   FAMILY HISTORY:
23   Unremarkable.

24   REVIEW OF SYSTEMS:
25   Negative.

26   PHYSICAL EXAMINATION:
27   Physical examination reveals a white female, slightly
28   overweight, in no apparent distress. Head, eyes, ears,
29   nose, and throat are **normocephalic** and **atraumatic**. The
30   lungs are clear to **auscultation**. Breasts are without
31   masses. The rectal examination is **guaiac negative** with
32   no masses. The abdomen is soft and slightly tender
33   to palpation in the right upper quadrant.

PATIENT: Sylvia Dos Santos
CHART #:
Page 2

34   RECOMMENDATION:
35   The patient should be admitted to the hospital for
36   further evaluation and possible **cholecystectomy**.

37   _____
38   Angela Rizzio, MD

39   AR/urs

40   d: 10/24/–
41   t: 10/25/–   Word Count 230
42   ▂▂   HPEGASSD.2

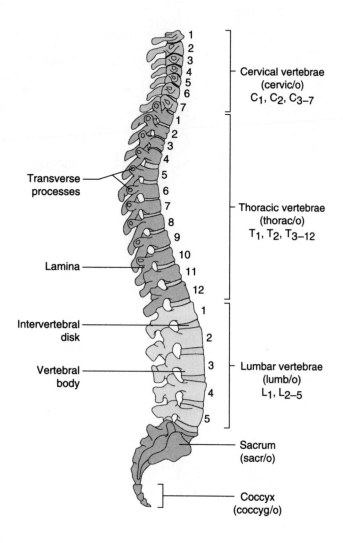

Cervical vertebrae
(cervic/o)
C_1, C_2, C_{3-7}

Transverse
processes

Thoracic vertebrae
(thorac/o)
T_1, T_2, T_{3-12}

Lamina

Intervertebral
disk

Vertebral
body

Lumbar vertebrae
(lumb/o)
L_1, L_{2-5}

Sacrum
(sacr/o)

Coccyx
(coccyg/o)

Spinal column

postpartum	After childbirth.
retrorectal	Behind, in back of the rectum.
sacrococcygeal	Concerning the sacrum and coccyx.
teratoma	Congenital tumor containing one or more of the three primary embryonic germ layers (hair and teeth may be present).
coccygectomy	Surgical excision of coccyx.
sacrectomy	Surgical excision of sacrum.
necrotic	Dead tissue.
histology	Study of the microscopic structure of tissue.
adenocarcinoma	Malignant tumor from a glandular organ.

HISTORY AND PHYSICAL EXAMINATION

1 PATIENT: Sofia Marine
2 CHART #:

3 HISTORY: The patient is a 33-year-old female school
4 teacher who is recently **postpartum** after having
5 delivered by C-section on 11/28/–.

6 On January 21, 20–, the patient underwent excision of
7 a **retrorectal** cystic mass described as a **sacrococcygeal**
8 **teratoma**. The operation consisted of a **coccygectomy**,
9 partial **sacrectomy** and dissection of a retrorectal
10 tumor. At the time, she was found to have **necrotic**
11 contents within this cystic mass, and the **histology**
12 revealed an **adenocarcinoma** arising in this "hindgut cyst."

13 Smears of the fluid surrounding the retrorectal tumor
14 at the time of operation (40 ml of bloody opaque fluid)
15 revealed malignant cells consistent with
16 adenocarcinoma. The background revealed extensive
17 necrosis.

18 PAST HISTORY: The patient is in, otherwise, good
19 health and does not see a doctor regularly for any
20 chronic medical illness. Her recent surgery was
21 performed by Dr. Leo Adams. The patient does not take
22 any medications. She does take a high-potency
23 B-vitamin with C, prenatal vitamins, etc. Other than the
24 C-section on 11/28/– and the current operation, she
25 has had no other surgery. She is allergic to
26 sulfonamides and codeine. She does not smoke or drink.
27 Her father died of Alzheimer's disease at the age of
28 61. Her mother is alive. A paternal aunt and
29 grandmother had colon cancer.

30 PHYSICAL EXAMINATION: Physical examination reveals
31 a healthy appearing female in no acute distress. Her
32 head, eyes, ears, nose, and throat are unremarkable.
33 There is no supraclavicular adenopathy. Lungs and
34 heart were not examined. Her liver is not enlarged to
35 palpation or percussion. The abdomen is soft, flat,
36 and nontender. There is no organomegaly or masses.
37 Inguinal regions are normal. There is a midline
38 incision from the posterior aspect of the anal orifice
39 to the sacrum which is well healed. Digital rectal
40 examination reveals the absence of a coccyx but is
41 otherwise normal. There are no perirectal or extra-rectal
42 masses either posteriorly or laterally. Anteriorly, a vaginal
43 examination is entirely within normal limits.

44   IMPRESSION:
45   1. Hindgut cyst with adenocarcinoma.

46   2. Malignant fluid in the surrounding tissue.

47   RECOMMENDATIONS: The patient is advised to undergo
48   pelvic radiation therapy with chemotherapy. There is
49   no current role for an operation in her clinical
50   situation.

51   _____
52   Cynthia Dean-Jamisson, MD

53   CDJ/urs

54   d: 2/3/—
55   t: 2/3/—   Word Count 395
56   🔲   HPEGASSM.3

HPEGASBS.4	Bella Stanford	Terminology Preview
asymptomatic		Showing no disease symptoms.
colonoscopy		Endoscopic examination of the colon, either transabdominally (relating to through or across the abdomen or abdominal wall) during laparotomy, or transanally (relating to through or across the anus or outer rectal opening) by means of a colonoscope.
embolism		Blood clot.
phlebitis		Inflammation of a vein.
supraclavicular adenopathy		Above the clavicle. Glandular disease.
palpation		Process of examining by application of the hands or fingers to the external surface of the body to detect evidence of disease or abnormalities in the various organs.
percussion		Use of the fingertips to tap the body lightly but sharply to determine position, size, and consistency of an underlying structure and the presence of fluid or pus in a cavity.
organomegaly		Enlargement of the viscera.
multinodulated		Having many nodules.
adenocarcinoma		Malignant tumor from a glandular organ.
cardiac catheterization		A long, fine catheter is passed through a peripheral blood vessel into the chambers of the heart under fluoroscopic control.

PUNCTUATION REFERENCES

Line 3	hyphen—compound modifier, Rule 1
Line 6	apostrophe—singular possessive, Rule 1
Line 10	semicolon—two independent clauses with one or more clauses containing a comma
Lines 10, 11	commas—parenthetical, Rule 10
Line 13	commas—parenthetical, Rule 10
Lines 15, 16	commas—parenthetical, Rule 10
Line 16	hyphen—compound modifier, Rule 1
Line 17	hyphen—compound modifier, Rule 1
Line 19	commas—parenthetical, Rule 10

Line 25	comma—conjunction, Rule 3
Line 26	comma—conjunction, Rule 3
Line 29	comma—two modifiers, Rule 2
Line 29	hyphen—compound modifier, Rule 1
Line 30	commas—series, Rule 1
Lines 33, 34	commas—series, Rule 1
Line 36	comma—parenthetical, Rule 10
Line 50	comma—introductory, Rule 7
Line 53	comma—introductory, Rule 7
Line 54	semicolon—two independent clauses with one or more clauses containing a comma
Line 55	comma—introductory, Rule 7

HISTORY AND PHYSICAL EXAMINATION

1   PATIENT: Bella Stanford
2   CHART #:

3   HISTORY: The patient is a 68-year-old retired female
4   who is **asymptomatic** with the exception of a known
5   history of angina pectoris.

6   The patient's physician performed a blood test and
7   found that she was anemic. He recommended appropriate
8   GI endoscopy and a barium enema. No tumors associated
9   with the GI blood loss were revealed. **Colonoscopy** was
10   requested; and this procedure, performed by Dr. Nathan
11   Jackson, revealed a large mass in the cecum or ascending
12   colon.

13   The patient is in, otherwise, reasonable health. She
14   sees Dr. Ventulous for the management of heart disease
15   characterized by angina pectoris. She takes Inderal,
16   80 mg, and uses a 40-mg nitro patch once daily. She
17   also takes cod-liver oil and Vitamin E.

18   PAST HISTORY: The patient underwent two breast
19   biopsies, one in 19– and one in 19–, and a
20   thyroidectomy in 19–. She has never been admitted to
21   a hospital for any major medical illness.

22   She is not allergic to any medication. She does not
23   smoke or drink. Her mother died of an **embolism**
24   following an operation for adhesions. Her father died
25   from **phlebitis**, but this is not clear. Her family
26   history of cancer is not clear, but she states that her
27   mother died at Brookside Hospital.

28   PHYSICAL EXAMINATION: Physical examination reveals a
29   well-developed, well-nourished female in no acute
30   distress. Head, eyes, ears, nose and throat are
31   unremarkable. There is no **supraclavicular adenopathy**.
32   Lungs and heart were not examined. Liver is not
33   enlarged to **palpation** or **percussion**. Abdomen is soft,
34   flat, and nontender. There is no **organomegaly** or
35   masses. Inguinal regions are normal. Rectal
36   examination, after the barium enema, reveals no
37   evidence of a filling defect or mass.

38   A telephone call to Dr. Jackson revealed that there was
39   an approximate 4 cm **multinodulated** mass in the cecum
40   consistent with a large polyp or an **adenocarcinoma**
41   causing the clinical anemia.

42 IMPRESSION:
43 1. Villus adenoma of the cecum and ascending colon
44   with secondary anemia.

45 2. Angina pectoris.

46 RECOMMENDATION: The patient is referred to
47 Dr. Amanda Joyce for preoperative medical evaluation.
48 An appropriate **cardiac catheterization** should be
49 scheduled in order to assess and possibly to treat her
50 angina. Once her coronary artery status is known, an
51 operation can be scheduled.

52 The patient was asked to obtain her colonoscopy report
53 and slides. In the presence of documentation, another
54 colonoscopy will not be necessary; but in the absence of
55 documentation, the patient will be scheduled to undergo
56 another colonoscopy on the day prior to the operation.

57   _____
58   J. Warren Higgins, MD

59 JWH/urs

60 d: 3/22/–
61 t: 3/23/–   Word Count 437
62   HPEGASBS.4

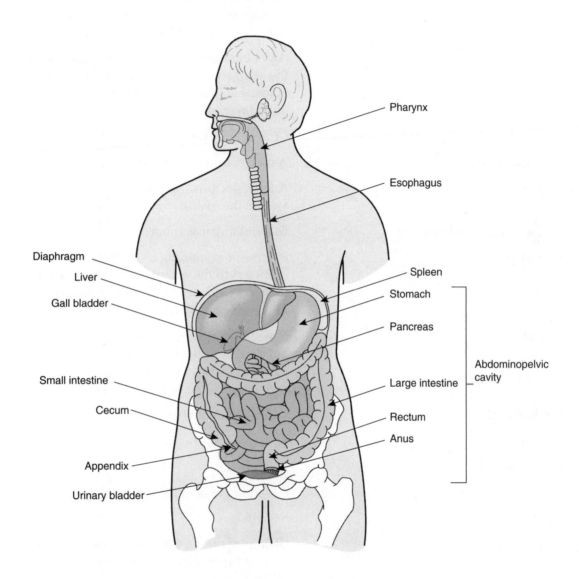

Organs of digestion and elimination

tenesmus	Spasmodic contraction of anal or vesical sphincter with pain and persistent desire to empty bowel or bladder with involuntary straining efforts.
colonoscopy	Endoscopic examination of the colon, either transabdominally during laparotomy, or transanally by means of a colonoscope.
epidermoid	Any tumor occurring at a noncutaneous (not at the skin) site and formed by inclusion of epidermal (pertaining to the cuticle or outer layer of skin) cells.
exophytic	Growing outward.
adenocarcinoma	A malignant tumor arising from a glandular organ.
angina	Angina pectoris (severe pain and constriction around the heart).
supraclavicular adenopathy	Glandular disease above the clavicle.
palpation	Process of examining by application of the hands or fingers to the external surface of the body to detect evidence of disease or abnormalities in the various organs.
percussion	Use of the fingertips to tap the body lightly but sharply to determine position, size, and consistency of an underlying structure and the presence of fluid or pus in a cavity.
organomegaly	Enlargement of visceral organs.
anteriorly	Referring to the abdominal side of the body.
circumferential	Encircling.
anorectal	Pertaining to both the anus and rectum.
squamous	Scalelike.
villus adenoma	Glandular tumor, filamentous (threadlike) process (outgrowth of membrane).
perineal	Concerning or situated on the perineum (pelvic floor).

HISTORY AND PHYSICAL EXAMINATION

1   PATIENT: James Kirkland
2   CHART #:

3   HISTORY: The patient is a 66-year-old retired male who
4   first noticed difficulty approximately eight months ago
5   with a change in bowel habits and "piles." His bowel
6   habits became more infrequent from moving his bowels
7   once daily to once every two or three days. A
8   protrusion was attributed to a hemorrhoid. Five to six
9   months ago, he began to notice bleeding. Three to four
10   months ago he noticed a flattening of his stool and
11   the onset of straining without a bowel movement, i.e.,
12   **tenesmus**. He now has a sense of incomplete defecation
13   and the presence of mucus in his stool. The patient
14   notes a 20-pound weight loss over the last 12 months.
15   He said there is no change in his appetite.

16   A **colonoscopy** was performed by Dr. Pailo, and the
17   patient was found to have a rectal tumor.

18   The patient underwent five biopsies. Surgical biopsy
19   No. 616 reveals **epidermoid** carcinoma and is,
20   undoubtedly, taken from an **exophytic** extra anal mass.
21   Biopsy No. 788 reveals an infiltrating **adenocarcinoma**
22   and biopsies No. 715 a, b, and c reveal either a polyp
23   or cancer arising inside the polyp.

24   The patient is in, otherwise, average health with
25   management of hypertension. He takes Isoptin, 240 mg,
26   and Hygroton. He also takes Kaon elixir, a
27   multivitamin, and iron tablets twice daily. He has no
28   major problems with any vessels.

29   PAST HISTORY: In 19–, he was admitted to the hospital
30   with **angina**. He was found on catheterization to have a
31   coronary thrombosis. Since that time, he has had no
32   chest pain at all. He is not allergic to any
33   medication and no longer smokes. He did smoke for 40
34   years from 19– to 19–. He has three alcoholic drinks
35   per day. His mother died of lobar pneumonia at the age
36   of 33. His father died at the age of 71 of heart disease.

37   PHYSICAL EXAMINATION: The patient is a well-developed,
38   well-nourished male in no acute distress. Head, eyes,
39   ears, nose, and throat are unremarkable. There is no
40   **supraclavicular adenopathy**. Lungs and heart were not
41   examined. Liver is not enlarged to **palpation** or

42   **percussion**. Abdomen is soft, flat, and nontender.
43   There are no masses or **organomegaly**. Inguinal regions
44   are normal. Rectal examination reveals the presence of
45   at least two distinct tumors. There is an exophytic
46   extra anal mass which is consistent with either a
47   perianal or an anal epidermoid carcinoma. I see no
48   component crossing the dented line. Digital rectal
49   examination reveals that the rectum is carpeted by a
50   mass which has thickened the wall of the rectum
51   **anteriorly**. The majority of the mass is
52   **circumferential**. The anterior plains between the tumor
53   and the prostate are intact but somewhat more difficult
54   to discern than usual. The lesion is nearly
55   circumferential. There is no margin between the tumor
56   and the **anorectal** junction, i.e., the dented line or
57   anal canal.

58   The slides are reviewed, and they reveal epidermoid
59   carcinoma (**squamous**) in the external lesion and
60   invasive adenocarcinoma in the rectal lesion.

61   IMPRESSION:
62   1. Adenocarcinoma of the rectum, primary, arising in a
63   **villus adenoma**.

64   2. Epidermoid carcinoma, probably perianal as opposed to
65   anal, but quite a sizable lesion of approximately 4 cm.

66   RECOMMENDATIONS:
67   1. The patient is advised to undergo combined radiation and
68   chemotherapy followed by abdominal **perineal** resection
69   with pelvic sidewall dissection.

70   2. The patient is referred to Dr. Smithson and
71   Dr. Perez for treatment.

72
73   Katherine T. Formatti, MD

74   KTF/urs

75   d: 4/17/—
76   t: 4/17/—   Word Count 582
77   HPEGASJK.5

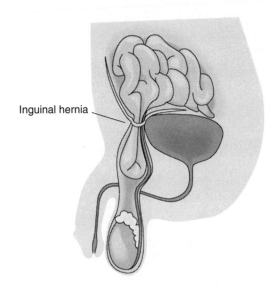

Inguinal hernia

Inguinal hernia

inguinal herniorrhaphy	Surgical repair of a hernia in the groin with suture of the abdominal wall.
erythema	Redness of the skin caused by congestion of the capillaries in the lower layers of the skin.
varicoceles	Varicosity (condition of a swollen or twisted vein) of the pampiniform plexus (a mesh of spermatic veins; network of nerves supplying the testicles) of the spermatic cord, forming a scrotal swelling.
guaiac	An alcoholic solution of guaiac (a tree resin) used for testing for occult blood in feces.

HISTORY AND PHYSICAL EXAMINATION

1   PATIENT: Gordon Mayerson

2   CHART #:

3   HISTORY: This is an 81-year-old attorney who noted

4   that a left groin bulge he had for the last five or six

5   years was increasing slowly in size. He denies any

6   abdominal pain, nausea, vomiting, or change in bowel

7   habits. He is on no medications.

8   PAST MEDICAL/SURGICAL HISTORY: Right **inguinal**

9   **herniorrhaphy**; tonsillectomy and adenoidectomy as

10   a child.

11   SOCIAL HISTORY: The patient smokes 10 cigarettes per

12   day. He has three children and six grandchildren.

13   PHYSICAL EXAMINATION: Head, eyes, ears, nose and

14   throat examination is unremarkable. Chest: Clear. Heart:

15   S1, S2. Abdomen: Flat, soft, nontender, nondistended,

16   normoactive bowel sounds. Genitalia: Within normal limits,

17   male uncircumcised. Large left hernia, easily reduced,

18   nontender, overlying skin intact with **erythema**. Bilateral

19   **varicoceles** present. No testicular masses. Rectal: Good

20   sphincter tone, large perianal skin tags. Prostate

21   moderately enlarged without masses, **guaiac** negative.

22   Neurological examination was without focality.

23   LABORATORY EXAMINATION: Within normal limits.

24   RECOMMENDATION: Admit this patient to the hospital for

25   surgery of left inguinal hernia.

26

27   Isaiah S. Price, MD

28   ISP/urs

29   d: 3/12—

30   t: 3/13—　 Word Count 197

31   ▄▄　 HPEGENGM.1

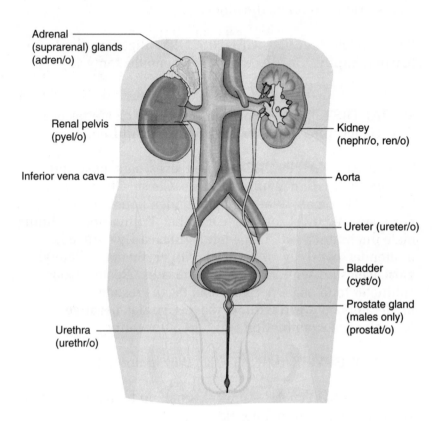

Adrenal
(suprarenal) glands
(adren/o)

Renal pelvis
(pyel/o)

Inferior vena cava

Urethra
(urethr/o)

Kidney
(nephr/o, ren/o)

Aorta

Ureter (ureter/o)

Bladder
(cyst/o)

Prostate gland
(males only)
(prostat/o)

Urinary system

flank	Part of body between ribs and upper border of ilium.
colicky	Painful spasm.
tonsillectomy	Excision of tonsils.
adenoidectomy	Excision of adenoids.
sphincter	Circular muscle that closes the anus, the external one being of striated muscle, the internal one, of plain muscle.
nephrolithiasis	Presence of calculi (commonly called stones composed of mineral salts; blockage of flow of urine from kidney if the ureter is blocked by the stones) in the kidney.

HISTORY AND PHYSICAL EXAMINATION

1   PATIENT: Leonard Nober

2   CHART #:

3   HISTORY: This is a 33-year-old male who complains of

4   right **flank** pain radiating to the right testicle. The

5   patient was well until one day prior to admission when

6   he states that he felt severe pain in the right flank

7   radiating to the groin. The pain awoke him from sleep.

8   The pain was **colicky** in nature, waxing and waning.

9   He noted no gross changes in the color of his urine.

10   PAST MEDICAL HISTORY: Unremarkable.

11   PAST SURGICAL HISTORY: **Tonsillectomy**, **adenoidectomy**

12   as a child.

13   ALLERGIES: No known allergies.

14   SOCIAL HISTORY: The patient has smoked three to five

15   packs of cigarettes daily for the past 20 years.

16   He has one to two alcoholic drinks a day. He has a

17   history of intravenous drug abuse.

18   FAMILY HISTORY: Significant in that the patient's

19   mother has had kidney stones.

20   PHYSICAL EXAMINATION: The patient is a well-developed,

21   well-nourished male, in no acute distress. He is alert

22   and oriented ×3. The head, ears, eyes, nose and

23   throat examination was within normal limits. The neck

24   is supple with a full range of motion. The chest is

25   clear. The heart has a regular rhythm. The abdomen is

26   soft and nontender, bowel sounds are present. Rectal

27   examination reveals no masses. **Sphincter** tone is good.

28   Stool is not present. There is no tenderness on

29   rectal examination.

30   Extremities: The right and left upper extremity had

31   multiple small healed burn wounds; otherwise full range

32   of motion.

33   Neurologically, the patient is intact with no deficits.

PATIENT: Leonard Nober
CHART #:
Page 2

34   RECOMMENDATION: Admit this patient for further
35   examination and evaluation for possible
36   **nephrolithiasis**.

37   _____
38   James T. Tsai, MD

39   JTT/urs

40   d: 8/6/—
41   t: 8/6/—   Word Count 291
42   ▣   HPEGENLN.2

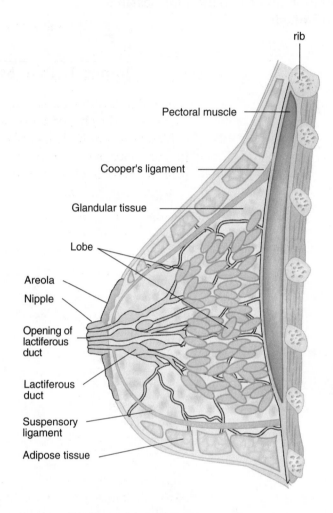

rib

Pectoral muscle

Cooper's ligament

Glandular tissue

Lobe

Areola

Nipple

Opening of
lactiferous
duct

Lactiferous
duct

Suspensory
ligament

Adipose tissue

Sagittal section of female breast

mammogram	A radiograph of the breast.
biopsy	Removal and examination, usually microscopic, of tissue from the living body.
rigors	Chills.
edema	Accumulation of fluid in a body part.
GI	Gastrointestinal.
renal	Pertaining to the kidney.
diabetes mellitus	A disorder of carbohydrate metabolism, characterized by hyperglycemia (increase of blood sugar as in diabetes) and glycosuria (the presence of glucose in the urine) and resulting from inadequate production or utilization of insulin.
D&C	Dilation and curettage (a surgical procedure that expands the cervical canal of the uterus [dilation] so that the surface lining of the uterine wall can be scraped [curettage]).
carcinoma	A new growth or malignant tumor that occurs in epithelial tissue; cancer.
PT	Prothrombin time (a test of clotting time made by determining the time for clotting to occur after thromboplastin and calcium are added to decalcified plasma; test is used to evaluate the effect of administration of anticoagulant drugs).
PTT	Partial thromboplastin (the third blood coagulation factor, factor III) time.
Qwave	A downward or negative wave of an electrocardiogram following the P wave. It is usually not prominent and may be absent without significance.
V_1	Placement position of a precordial (pertaining to the precordium or epigastrium. The area on the anterior surface of the body overlying the heart and the lower part of the thorax) lead on fourth intercostal space (space between the ribs) at right sternal border for an electrocardiogram.
Tspine	Thoracic spine (consisting of 12 thoracic vertebrae) between the cervical and lumbar spinal areas.

HISTORY AND PHYSICAL EXAMINATION

1   PATIENT: Ann Quickens
2   CHART #:

3   HISTORY:
4   The patient is an 82-year-old female who reported that
5   a right breast shadow was found on a **mammogram**
6   performed one month ago.

7   The patient was seen by Dr. Wong approximately one week
8   ago, and Dr. Wong recommended that she have a **biopsy** of
9   the right breast mass.

10   The patient denied any recent fevers, chills, **rigors**,
11   arm **edema**, breast pain, dimpling or deformity of
12   nipple, discharge, or previous breast masses.

13   PAST MEDICAL HISTORY:
14   The patient denied any history of pulmonary, peptic
15   ulcer, **GI**, **renal**, cardiac, or coronary artery disease.
16   The patient may have had some questionable history
17   of **diabetes mellitus**, however.

18   PAST SURGICAL HISTORY:
19   The patient had an appendectomy seven years ago for a
20   ruptured appendix and a **D&C** 10 years ago without
21   complications.

22   SOCIAL HISTORY:
23   The patient denied smoking, alcohol, or drug use.

24   MEDICATIONS:
25   None.

26   ALLERGIES:
27   None.

28   FAMILY HISTORY:
29   Negative family history of **carcinoma**.

30   REVIEW OF SYSTEMS:
31   Noncontributory.

32   PHYSICAL EXAM:
33   Blood pressure 150/80, pulse 80, respirations 14. In
34   general, the patient was a well-developed,
35   well-nourished female in no apparent distress. Her
36   physical was significant only for her right breast mass
37   which was palpated. No axillary adenopathy was noted.

PATIENT: Ann Quickens
CHART #:
Page 2

38 LABORATORY:
39 Hemoglobin/hematocrit 11.6/37.5, white blood cell count
40 of 6.1, platelet count 250, sodium 145, chloride 106,
41 bicarbonate 24, glucose 118, BUN/creatinine 28.0/1.3,
42 **PT/PTT** 11.8/24.0.

43 EKG: Normal sinus rhythm. Normal axis. No acute
44 changes. However, possible **Qwave** was noted in V_1.
45 Chest x-ray: Normal heart, no infiltrates or effusions
46 were noted. **Tspine**: Degenerative changes were
47 present on chest film.

48 RECOMMENDATION:
49 The patient should be admitted to the hospital for
50 further evaluation and possible mastectomy of
51 right breast.

52 _____
53 John K. Montesinos, MD

54 JKM/urs

55 d: 11/28/–
56 t: 11/29/– Word Count 303
57 HPEINTAQ.1

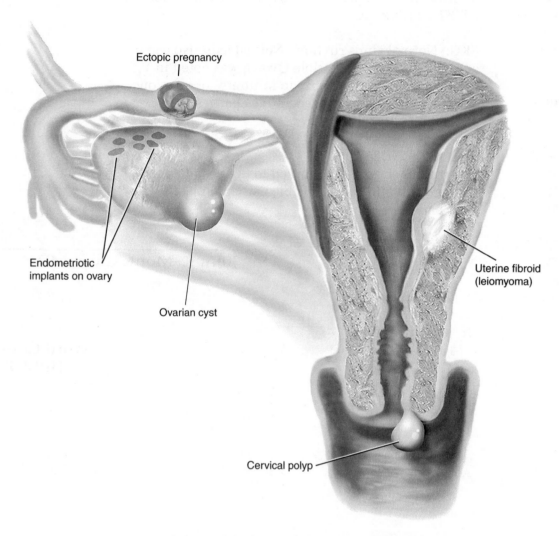

Ectopic pregnancy

Endometriotic
implants on ovary

Ovarian cyst

Uterine fibroid
(leiomyoma)

Cervical polyp

Pathology of the female reproductive system

tubal ligation	Binding or tying off of the fallopian tubes.
ectopic pregnancy	Implantation of the fertilized ovum outside of the uterine cavity.
dorsum	Back or posterior surface of a part.
PIP	Proximal interphalangeal (joint) (pertaining to the center of a joint between two fingers or toes).
subcutaneous	Beneath the skin.
distal	Remote, farther from any point of reference.
flexion	The act of bending, or the condition of being bent.
abduction	The lateral movement of the limbs away from the median plane of the body.

HISTORY AND PHYSICAL EXAMINATION

1 PATIENT: Gloria Ward
2 CHART #:

3 HISTORY: This patient is a 35-year-old right-handed
4 female who sustained injury to her left thumb on
5 August 13, 20– while opening a jar at home. The patient
6 came to the emergency room with no other injury, no
7 history of hand surgery, or injury in the past.

8 PAST HISTORY: Essentially unremarkable. No
9 hypertension, no diabetes, no coronary artery disease,
10 and no cancer.

11 PAST SURGICAL HISTORY: **Tubal ligation** and **ectopic**
12 **pregnancy**.

13 SOCIAL HISTORY: The patient is a single female who
14 smokes a half pack of cigarettes a day and drinks
15 alcohol socially. The patient was noted to be
16 extremely anxious and quite uncooperative with the
17 staff. She admitted to long use of cocaine.

18 PHYSICAL EXAMINATION: Chest was clear bilaterally.
19 Heart had a regular rate and rhythm. Abdomen was soft
20 and nontender; there was a lower abdominal healed scar.
21 Rectal examination was nontender; there were no masses.
22 Breasts were symmetrical and nontender with
23 no discharge.

24 Examination of her extremities revealed a single,
25 3 to 4 cm curved laceration on the **dorsum** of the left
26 thumb at the level of the **PIP** joint with
27 **subcutaneous** tissue exposed with no gross tendon
28 lacerations. There was no active bleeding.

29 Neurosensory examination was intact with good **distal**
30 capillary refill. She had full **flexion** but decreased
31 strength on extension. Questionable decreased strength
32 on **abduction** of the hand was noted.

33 There were no other injuries. Her preliminary x-rays
34 showed no fracture.

35 IMPRESSION: Hand laceration with possible tendon injury.

36   RECOMMENDATION: Admit the patient to the hospital for
37   further evaluation of possible tendon injury.

38   _____
39   Gale T. Peters, MD

40   GTP/urs

41   d: 8/14/—
42   t: 8/14/—   Word Count 291
43   ▟▙   HPEMUSGW.1

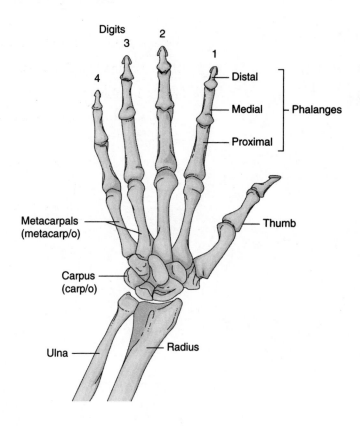

Bones of the hand

proximal phalanx	A finger bone that articulates with a metacarpal bone with the center of the body as the point of reference.
GI	Gastrointestinal.
afebrile	Without a fever.
extraocular	Outside the eye.
icterus	Jaundice.
sclerae	White fibrous tissue of the eyes.
lymphadenopathy	Disease of the lymph nodes.
submental	Under the chin.
auscultation	Percussion (process of listening for sounds within the body).
cyanosis	Slightly bluish or dark purple due to reduced hemoglobin in the blood.
edema	Accumulation of excess fluid in a body cavity.
comminuted fracture	Fracture in which the bone is broken or splintered into pieces.

HISTORY AND PHYSICAL EXAMINATION

1   PATIENT: Jane Brost

2   CHART #:

3   HISTORY:

4   The patient is a 31-year-old female who fractured the

5   **proximal phalanx** of her fourth or ring finger on her

6   right dominant hand. She never had had an injury to

7   this extremity, nor had she had any prior surgery to

8   the hand.

9   The injury occurred while she was walking her dog. The

10   dog's leash was wrapped around her finger. The dog was

11   startled by a loud noise and began to run and severely

12   pulled on the leash wrapped around her finger. As a

13   result, the finger was fractured.

14   PAST HISTORY:

15   She had a horseback injury at the age of 16. She suffered

16   a temporary loss of consciousness after the fall and

17   a small skull fracture. Medically, though, she has

18   no past medical history, no diabetes, no heart disease,

19   no hypertension, and no **GI** dysfunction.

20   ALLERGIES:

21   None.

22   MEDICATIONS:

23   None.

24   SOCIAL HISTORY:

25   The patient is a writer and has published a few works.

26   She drinks alcohol socially and does not smoke

27   cigarettes or take any unprescribed drugs.

28   REVIEW OF SYSTEMS:

29   Noncontributory.

30   PHYSICAL EXAMINATION:

31   Exam revealed a pleasant, well-developed female in no

32   acute distress. Vital signs were stable, and she was

33   **afebrile**. Head and neck exam was normal. **Extraocular**

34   movements were intact. No **icterus** was noted in the

35   **sclerae**. The patient had no **lymphadenopathy** in the

36   **submental** or cervical region.

37 Heart exam was normal with no murmurs noted. Breasts
38 were without masses or lesions. Lungs were clear to
39 **auscultation**. Abdomen was flat and soft with positive
40 bowel sounds. No gross masses were noted. Rectal was
41 heme negative. No masses or lesions were palpated.

42 Extremities: Essentially normal without clubbing,
43 **cyanosis**, or **edema**.

44 X-rays revealed a badly **comminuted fracture** of the
45 right fourth finger with an articular extension.

46 NEUROLOGICAL EXAMINATION:
47 The patient was alert and oriented ×3. She was
48 neurologically intact. Cranial nerves were intact.

49 RECOMMENDATION:
50 Admit the patient to the hospital for surgical repair of the
51 comminuted fracture of the fourth finger of the right hand.

52 _____
53 Leona Davis, MD

54 LD/urs

55 d: 10/6/—
56 t: 10/6/—
57 �

Word Count 364
HPEMUSJB.2

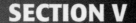

Special Procedures Reports

OVERVIEW

In this section the student will be transcribing special procedures reports specific to the cardio-vascular, endocrine, female reproductive, gastrointestinal, genitourinary, hematic, musculoskeletal, nervous, and respiratory body systems.

Terminology previews are provided for each report. Punctuation references illustrating uses of the comma, hyphen, colon, apostrophe, and period (placement of) are provided in seven reports.

SPECIAL PROCEDURES REPORTS

Special procedures reports include procedures such as magnetic resonance imaging (MRI), computerized axial tomography (CAT), and sonogram. These reports are customarily prepared by the office or department doing the procedure. The format will vary according to the office's or department's preference.

Use of a Macro

It is recommended that the student prepare a macro on a word processor to contain the word, PATIENT:. The macro can be named and retrieved with Alt x. (Consult your instruction manual for macro preparation, as needed.)

Multiple Page Headings

When the report exceeds one page, key a heading to include the patient's name and page number beginning on the first line of each succeeding page. For example,

> Barbara Bradley
>
> Page 2

Saving and Coding Transcripts

The student should name and save each transcribed report with the code provided at the end of each report.

INSTRUCTIONAL OBJECTIVES

In this chapter, the student will:

1. Transcribe special procedures reports of varying lengths in report format.
2. Learn terminology relative to the cardiovascular, endocrine, female reproductive, gastrointestinal, genitourinary, hematic, musculoskeletal, nervous, and respiratory body systems.
3. Reinforce understanding of the use of comma (series, conjunction, two-adjective modifier, parenthetical, introductory), hyphen (compound modifier and range of numbers), colon, and period (inside quotation marks).

REMINDERS: Preview highlighted medical terms and punctuation references in the report.
Listen to the tape to become familiar with it.
Transcribe the report inserting punctuation "cues."
Print out a hard copy.
Check carefully your transcribed report word by word to the text transcript.

THE TRANSCRIPT IN THE TEXT IS CHECKED <u>ONLY AFTER</u> YOU HAVE COMPLETED YOUR TRANSCRIPTION.

Record the number of lines transcribed and the number of minutes needed to complete the report.
Make corrections; submit the corrected transcript to your instructor.

SPECIAL PROCEDURES REPORTS INDEX

	Patient Name	Code Name	Word Count
CAR	AMIR BEKTESEVIK	SPCARAB.1	104
	BERNADETTE O'HARA	SPCARBO.2*	123
	LAWRENCE AIELLO	SPCARLA.3*	148
	BARBARA BRADLEY	SPCARBB.4*	563
END	MIRIAM GLEASON	SPENDMG.1	185
FEM	BARBARA MORGAN	SPFEMBM.1	143
	GLADYS TRENT	SPFEMGT.2*	227
	THERESA ALLENBY	SPFEMTA.3	268
GAS	FRED GRAUER	SPGASFG.7	105
	MARK SMITH	SPGASMS.8	205
	SAKURA NWOKE	SPGASSN.9	207
GEN	GERALD OLSEN	SPGENGO.1	66
	CLIFFORD BARTON	SPGENCB.2*	77
	HARRY COHEN	SPGENHC.3	124
	DANIELLE CAPUTO	SPGENDC.4	155
HEM	TOM CLARKE	SPHEMTC.1	121
MUS	SALLY BLUMBERG	SPMUSSB.1	81
	VIOLET DONG	SPMUSVD.3	138
	ANN MORGAN	SPMUSAM.4	139
	ROBERT GATTI	SPMUSRG.7*	174
	DANIEL FERBER	SPMUSDF.9	210
NER	KATHY CRUZ	SPNERKC.1	98
	FELIX GREENE	SPNERFG.2	121
	DONALD ERCOLANO	SPNERDE.3	139
	JENNIFER MARTIN	SPNERJM.4*	151
	PETER SMYTH	SPNERPS.5	164
	ANTHONY FERRARA	SPNERAF.6	169
RES	ARIEL EUSEBIO	SPRESAE.1	84
	BARRY AHRENS	SPRESBA.2	148

*Punctuation References

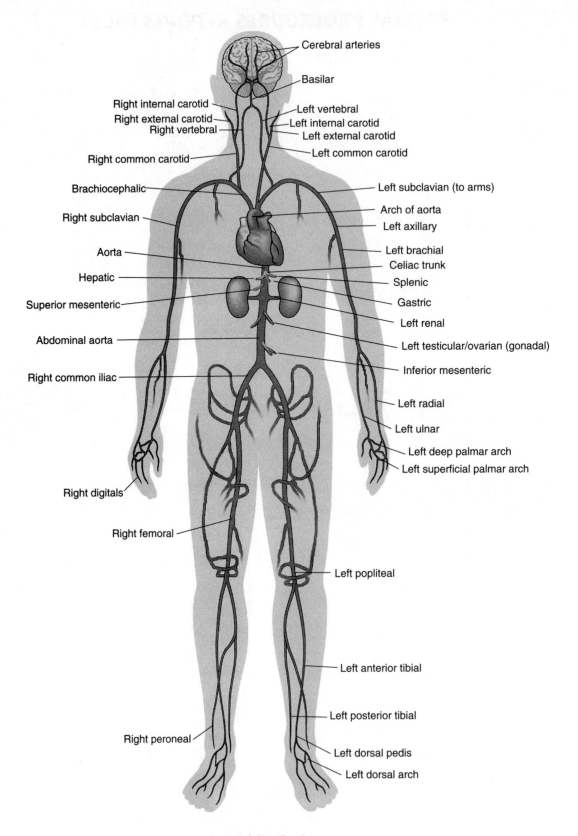

Arterial distribution

arteriogram	A radiograph of an artery.
carotid	Relating to the carotid artery, the principal artery of the neck.
distal	Remote; farther from any point of reference.
opacified	Impenetrable by visible light rays or by other forms of radiant energy such as x-rays.
patent	Open, unobstructed, or not closed.
endarterectomy	Excision of thickened atheromatous (pertaining to fatty degeneration or thickening of the walls of the larger arteries occurring in atherosclerosis) areas of the innermost coat of an artery.
stenosis	Narrowing or contraction of a body passage or opening.

INTRAOPERATIVE RIGHT **CAROTID ARTERIOGRAM**

1   PATIENT: Amir Bektesevik

2   Comparison is made with the preoperative study dated
3   May 26, 20–.

4   A single intraoperative right **carotid arteriogram** is
5   submitted for interpretation. The catheter tip is
6   located in the **distal** common carotid artery.
7   The injection has **opacified** a widely **patent**
8   **endarterectomy** site. The prior **stenosis** located at the
9   origin of the right internal carotid artery has been
10 completely reduced. The right internal carotid artery
11 is widely patent into the intracranial circulation.
12 The external carotid artery is also widely patent.

13 IMPRESSION: Intraoperative arteriogram demonstrating
14 a widely patent right carotid endarterectomy site.

15 _____

16 Issuance Astigmias, MD

17 IA/urs

18 d: 4/16/–
19 t: 4/16/–   Word Count 104
20 ▣   SPCARAB.1

distal		Remote; farther from any point of reference.
bifurcation		A division into two branches.
endarterectomy		Excision of thickened atheromatous areas of the innermost coat of an artery.
patent		Open, unobstructed, or not closed.
opacification		The development of an opacity.

PUNCTUATION REFERENCES

| Line 9 | commas—parenthetical, Rule 10 |
| Line 10 | hyphen—range of numbers |

INTRAOPERATIVE LEFT CAROTID ANGIOGRAM

PATIENT: Bernadette O'Hara

Comparison is made with the preoperative study dated
June 29, 20–.

Injection has been made into the **distal** left common
carotid artery just proximal to the **bifurcation**. The
carotid **endarterectomy** site is widely **patent** with
complete **opacification** of the left internal carotid
artery into the intracranial circulation. The left
external carotid artery remains occluded, however, a
short 1–2 cm segment of this vessel is opacified on the
current study. The prior stenotic segment at the
origin of the left internal carotid artery is now
widely patent.

IMPRESSION:
1. Intraoperative left carotid arteriogram documenting
   a widely patent left common carotid and internal
   carotid artery endarterectomy site.

2. External carotid artery remains occluded.

_____

Matthew Long, MD

ML/urs

d: 7/16/–
t: 7/16/–
📼

Word Count 123
SPCARBO.2

SPCARLA.3	Lawrence Aiello	Terminology Preview
opacification		The development of an opacity.
bifurcation		A division into two branches.
endarterectomy		Excision of thickened atheromatous areas of the innermost coat of an artery.
stenosis		Narrowing or contraction of a body passage or opening.

PUNCTUATION REFERENCES

Line 5	comma—introductory phrase, Rule 7
Line 13	comma—introductory phrase, Rule 7

INTRAOPERATIVE RIGHT CAROTID ARTERIOGRAM

1   PATIENT: Lawrence Aiello

2   Comparison is made with the preoperative arteriogram
3   dated June 16, 20–.

4   Two radiographs have been submitted labeled #1 and #2.

5   On the initial radiograph, there is **opacification** of
6   the distal right common carotid artery **bifurcation** and
7   internal and external carotid arteries. The carotid
8   **endarterectomy** site is noted. At the margin of the
9   endarterectomy site in the proximal right internal
10   carotid artery a residual 50% **stenosis** is present.
11   This is at the site of the prior severe 95%
12   focal stenosis.

13   On the radiograph labeled #2, the endarterectomy site
14   is now widely patent with no significant stenosis
15   present in the right internal carotid artery. The
16   right internal carotid artery is widely patent into the
17   intracranial circulation. The external carotid artery
18   remains patent.

19   IMPRESSION: Intraoperative right carotid angiogram
20   documenting a carotid endarterectomy with the final
21   film demonstrating a widely patent result.

22   _____

23   Janice Lee, MD

24   JL/urs

25   d: 7/15/—
26   t: 7/15/—   Word Count 148
27   ▣   SPCARLA.3

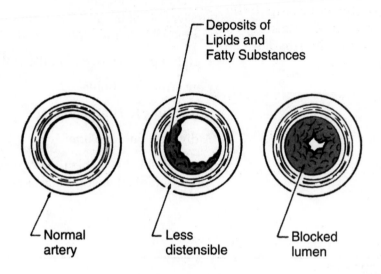

Deposits of
Lipids and
Fatty Substances

Normal
artery

Less
distensible

Blocked
lumen

Atherosclerosis of an artery

CABG	Coronary artery bypass graft.
claudication	Limping or lameness.
femoral	Pertaining to the femur or to the thigh.
atherosclerotic	A form of arteriosclerosis characterized by accumulation of fatty plaques in the arteries.
hemodynamically	Referring to a study of the forces involved in circulating blood through the body.
mesenteric	Referring to the peritoneal (concerning the peritoneum, the serous membrane reflected over the viscera and lining the abdominal cavity) fold encircling the greater part of the small intestine and connecting the intestine to the posterior abdominal wall.
hypogastric	Pertaining to the lower middle of the abdomen.
peroneal	Concerning the fibula.
tibioperoneal	Concerning the tibia and fibula.
bifurcation	A division into two branches.
opacified	Impenetrable by visible light rays or by other forms of radiant energy such as x-rays.

PUNCTUATION REFERENCES

Line 2	hyphens—compound modifier, Rule 1
Lines 3, 4	commas—series, Rule 1
Line 10	hyphen—number used with word as compound modifier
Line 11	hyphen—range of numbers
Line 13	hyphen—compound modifier, Rule 1
Line 19	comma—parenthetical, Rule 10
Line 26	commas—series, Rule 1
Lines 33, 35, 38	hyphen—compound modifier, Rule 1
Lines 66, 67	commas—parenthetical, Rule 10
Line 68	hyphen—compound modifier, Rule 1

DISTAL ABDOMINAL AORTOGRAM AND BILATERAL
LOWER EXTREMITY ARTERIOGRAM

1   PATIENT: Barbara Bradley

2   CLINICAL DATA: A 73-year-old woman with a long history
3   of tobacco use, non-insulin dependent diabetes
4   mellitus, status post **CABG**, hypertension, is now
5   admitted for evaluation of bilateral one block with left
6   slightly greater than right calf **claudication**. A
7   consult was placed in the chart.

8   A right common **femoral** artery puncture was performed
9   with standard Seldinger technique. Intravenous Versed
10   and Fentanyl were utilized for IV sedation. A 4-French
11   pigtail catheter was inserted and advanced to the L2–3
12   level. An abdominal aortogram and bilateral lower
13   extremity arteriogram with cut-film technique was
14   performed from this site.

15   The study is remarkable for a distal abdominal aorta
16   that is narrow in caliber measuring approximately
17   17 mm. Moderate **atherosclerotic** plaque is present in
18   the distal abdominal aorta. No focal stenosis in the
19   aorta is present, however.

20   A **hemodynamically** significant 80–90% focal stenosis is
21   present in the proximal right common iliac artery. A
22   75% focal stenosis is present at the origin of the left
23   common iliac artery. The inferior **mesenteric** artery is
24   patent and supplies prominent collateral vessels to the
25   pelvis via the hemorrhoidal arteries. The distal
26   common iliac arteries, external iliac arteries, and
27   **hypogastric** arteries are widely patent bilaterally.

28   Both common femoral arteries are widely patent as well
29   as the profunda femoris arteries. There is moderate
30   generalized atherosclerotic disease involving both
31   superficial femoral arteries and popliteal arteries. A
32   focal 50% stenosis is present at the transition of the
33   right superficial femoral artery to the above-knee
34   popliteal artery. A 90% focal stenosis is present at
35   this same site in the left SFA above-knee popliteal
36   artery. A 2 cm 75% stenotic segment is present in the
37   right popliteal artery at the level of the knee joint.

38 A focal 90% stenosis is present in the mid-left
39 popliteal artery.

40 There is single vessel runoff bilaterally via the
41 **peroneal** arteries. A severe 90% focal stenosis is
42 present in the proximal right **tibioperoneal** trunk. The
43 peroneal artery is then widely patent to its normal
44 **bifurcation** above the ankle. An anterior communicating
45 branch reconstitutes the distal segment of the right
46 anterior tibial artery. This vessel is not continuous
47 into the dorsalis pedis artery but rather gives off a
48 collateral vessel which then reconstitutes the distal
49 right dorsalis pedis artery. A posterior communicating
50 branch from the peroneal artery reconstitutes posterior
51 tarsal branches. The plantar arch is **opacified** in the
52 right foot.

53 The left peroneal artery is widely patent to above the
54 ankle where it gives off a collateral vessel that
55 reconstitutes the distal left anterior tibial artery.
56 This vessel is directly continuous into the dorsalis
57 pedis artery. No plantar arch was visualized in the
58 left foot as in the right foot.

59 The pigtail catheter was removed over a wire and
60 hemostasis obtained by compression. The patient
61 tolerated the procedure well and left the department in
62 good condition.

63 IMPRESSION:
64 1. Hemodynamically significant stenoses in both
65   common iliac arteries as described above.

66 2. Hemodynamically significant stenoses, left
67   greater than right, at the transition of
68   the SFA to above-knee popliteal artery
69   and in the midpopliteal arteries.

70 3. Single vessel runoff bilaterally via the
71   peroneal artery as described above. Focal
72   90% stenosis right tibioperoneal trunk.

Barbara Bradley
Page 3

IMPRESSION (continued):

73   4. Opacification of plantar arches in
74   both feet.

75   _____
76   Harvey Long, MD

77   HL/urs

78   d: 4/14/—
79   t: 4/14/—   Word Count 563
80   SPCARBB.4

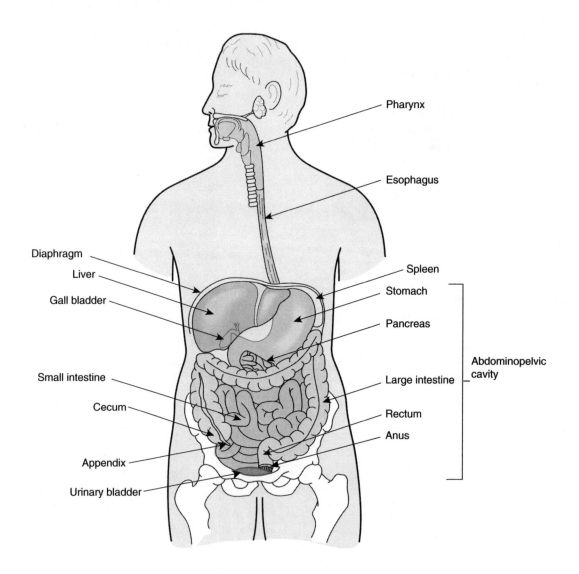

Gastrointestinal system

- Pharynx
- Esophagus
- Diaphragm
- Liver
- Gall bladder
- Spleen
- Stomach
- Pancreas
- Abdominopelvic cavity
- Small intestine
- Large intestine
- Cecum
- Rectum
- Anus
- Appendix
- Urinary bladder

subdiaphragmatic	Below the diaphragm.
pancreatectomy	Excision of the pancreas.
hepatic	Pertaining to the liver.
anterior	Situated at or directed toward the front.
percutaneous	Effected through the skin.
purulent	Containing or forming pus.
aspirated	Suctioned.

REPOSITIONING AND REPLACEMENT OF ANTERIOR
SUBDIAPHRAGMATIC ABSCESS DRAINAGE CATHETER

1   PATIENT: Miriam Gleason

2   CLINICAL DATA: The patient is status post total
3   **pancreatectomy** and has a **hepatic** abscess and an
4   **anterior** subdiaphragmatic abscess. The abcesses are
5   drained with a **percutaneous** catheter. A recent CT scan
6   was notable for an undrained collection, located
7   anteriorly, just beneath the diaphragm and anterior to
8   the liver.

9   Under fluoroscopic control, water-soluble contrast was
10 injected via the 16-French sump drainage catheter
11 located in the anterior subdiaphragmatic collection.

12 The more superior, undrained component of the
13 collection was opacified.

14 The prior drainage catheter was removed, and utilizing
15 a coaxial wire and catheter system, a new 16-French
16 nonlocking sump catheter was inserted with the distal
17 tip positioned within the more superior component of
18 the abscess. Approximately 100 cc of **purulent** material
19 was **aspirated**. The abscess catheter was irrigated, and
20 the catheter was sutured in place. The catheter was
21 attached to a gravity drainage bag. The patient
22 tolerated the procedure well and left the department in
23 good condition.

24 IMPRESSION: Repositioning and replacement of
25 16-French nonlocking sump drainage catheter into
26 anterior subdiaphragmatic abscess.

27 _____
28 Gloria Taverno, MD

29 GT/urs

30 d: 4/16/—
31 t: 4/16/—   Word Count 185
32 📼   SPENDMG.1

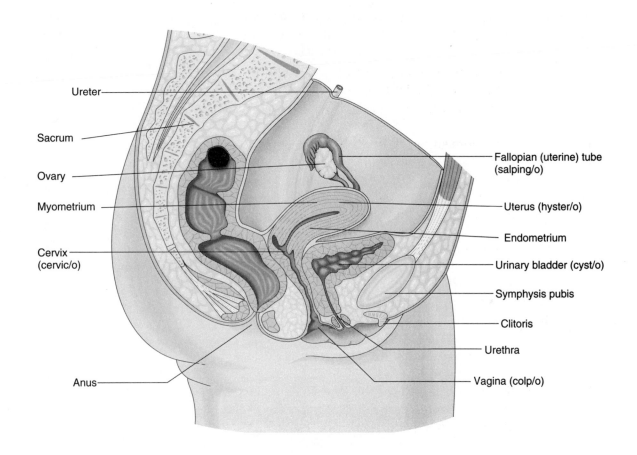

Ureter

Sacrum

Ovary

Myometrium

Cervix
(cervic/o)

Anus

Fallopian (uterine) tube
(salping/o)

Uterus (hyster/o)

Endometrium

Urinary bladder (cyst/o)

Symphysis pubis

Clitoris

Urethra

Vagina (colp/o)

Female reproductive system

fundal	Pertaining to the body of the uterus above the openings of the fallopian tubes.
endometrial	Pertaining to the endometrium (the mucous membrane lining the inner surface of the uterus).
nabothi cyst	Retention cyst formed by the nabothian glands at the neck of the uterus.
myoma	A tumor formed of muscle tissue.
leiomyosarcoma	A sarcoma (cancer arising from connective tissue, such as muscle or bone) containing cells of smooth muscle.

PELVIC SONOGRAM INCLUDING TRANSVAGINAL SCANNING

1   PATIENT: Barbara Morgan

2   The uterus is being displaced posteriorly by a large
3   uterine mass which measures approximately 10 cm
4   in length × 7.8 cm in depth × 9.8 cm in transverse
5   dimension.

6   This mass is solid but heterogeneous in echo texture
7   and appears to be extending into the abdominal cavity
8   from the **fundal** aspect of the uterus. The **endometrial**
9   echo within the uterus is enlarged. Some **nabothi cyst**
10   formation is noted in the cervical region.

11   Both ovaries are identified and are unremarkable. A
12   trace of free fluid is noted in the cul-de-sac.

13   IMPRESSION: Uterus displaced posteriorly by a
14   dominant large uterine mass with dimensions as
15   given above. Rule out **myoma/leiomyosarcoma**,
16   based on apparent rate of growth, for example.

17   _____
18   Samuel Davis, MD

19   SD/urs

20   d: 6/16/—
21   t: 6/16/—   Word Count 143
22   ▆▆   SPFEMBM.1

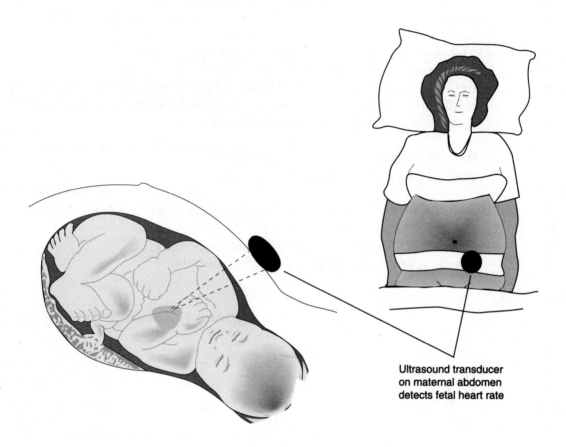

Placement of ultrasound transducer to detect fetal heart rate

Ultrasound transducer
on maternal abdomen
detects fetal heart rate

SPFEMGT.2	Gladys Trent	Terminology Preview
transabdominal		Across the abdominal wall or through the abdominal cavity.
singleton intrauterine gestation		The development of one infant within the uterus beginning with conception and culminating in birth.
transverse lie		The position of the long axis of the fetus lying from side to side with respect to that of the mother.
uterine		Pertaining to the uterus.
placenta		An organ that joins mother and offspring during pregnancy, acts as a nutrient storehouse, and helps nourish the fetus.
anterior		Situated at or directed toward the front; opposite of posterior.
amniotic		Pertaining to the amnion (a thin, transparent sac that holds the fetus suspended in the liquor amnii, or amniotic fluid).
fetal		Of or pertaining to a fetus or to the period of its development.
intracranial		Within the cranium.
biometry		The application of statistical methods to biological facts.
BPD		Biparietal (concerning two parietal bones that form the roof and sides of the skull) diameter (of fetal head).
umbilical		Pertaining to the umbilicus (navel).
systolic		Pertaining to systole (part of the heart cycle in which the heart is in contraction).
diastolic		Pertaining to diastole (part of the heart cycle in which the heart is in relaxation, alternating with systole or contraction).

PUNCTUATION REFERENCES

Lines 8, 9	commas—series, Rule 1
Line 8	hyphen—compound modifier, Rule 1
Line 10	comma—conjunction, Rule 3
Line 12	colon—Rule 1
Lines 13, 15, 17, 19	comma—separation of weeks and days
Line 24	apostrophe—plural possessive, Rule 2

OBSTETRICAL ULTRASOUND

1   PATIENT: Gladys Trent

2   **Transabdominal** ultrasound demonstrates a **singleton**
3   **intrauterine gestation** in **transverse lie**. The lower
4   **uterine** segment is normal. The **placenta** is **anterior**
5   and low lying. There is normal **amniotic** fluid volume.
6   **Fetal** cardiac activity is present.

7   Evaluation of fetal anatomy reveals normal **intracranial**
8   contents, a four-chamber heart, normal stomach,
9   kidneys, urinary bladder, spine and extremities. The
10   fetus was active during the examination, and it was
11   difficult to document the cord insertion.

12   **Biometry** is as follows: **BPD** measures 3.9 cm
13   corresponding to a gestational age of 18 weeks, 0 days.

14   The head circumference measures 15.0 cm corresponding
15   to a gestational age of 18 weeks, 0 days. The femur
16   length measures 2.7 cm corresponding to a gestational
17   age of 18 weeks, 1 day. The abdominal circumference
18   measures 12.9 cm corresponding to a gestational age of
19   18 weeks, 1 day.

20   Color duplex Doppler interrogation of the **umbilical**
21   artery reveals a peak **systolic** to **diastolic** ratio
22   of 2.5.

23   IMPRESSION: Singleton intrauterine gestation in
24   transverse lie at 18 weeks' gestation. Fetal anatomy
25   appears normal. The cord insertion was not
26   documented due to a highly active fetus. The
27   patient is requested to return at a time convenient
28   to her for documentation of a normal cord insertion.
29   This is offered to the patient at no additional charge.

30
31   Samuel Jordan, MD

32   SJ/urs

33   d: 4/13/—
34   t: 4/13/—
35   ▰

Word Count 227
SPFEMGT.2

gestational	Pertaining to gestation.
decidual	Pertaining to or resembling the decidua (endometrium or lining of the uterus during pregnancy, and the tissue around the ectopically located fertilized ovum, e.g., in the fallopian tube or peritoneal cavity).
myoma	A tumor formed of muscle tissue.
subserosal	Below a serous (producing or containing serum or a serumlike substance) membrane.
intramurally	Within the walls of a hollow organ or cavity.

OBSTETRIC SONOGRAM

1   PATIENT: Theresa Allenby

2   The uterus is markedly enlarged. Twin intrauterine gestations
3   are identified. Sac "A" refers to the sac on the right side, and
4   sac "B" to the sac on the left side.

5   Fetus A measures 1.6 cm in length corresponding to a maturity
6   of 8 weeks and 0 days with a 5-day variability. A yolk sac is
7   identified within this sac.

8   Fetus B measures 1.7 cm in length corresponding to a maturity
9   of 8 weeks and 1 day maturity with a 5-day variability.

10   Both **gestational** sacs show good **decidual** reaction and adequate
11   amniotic fluid. A thick septum is seen separating the two sacs.
12   Fetal cardiac motion is identified within both fetuses.

13   Three uterine fibroids are identified. Number 1 is in the lower
14   uterine segment/cervical area posteriorly and measures 3.7 cm
15   in length × 2.2 cm in depth. Number 2 lies above this, again in
16   the lower uterine segment and measures 3.8 cm in length × 3.2 cm
17   in depth. The largest one is Number 3 arising from the anterior lower
18   body of the uterus. This **myoma** measures 7.2 cm in length × 5.6 cm
19   in depth. This one is **subserosal** and extends **intramurally**. It is
20   causing a marked contour bulge of the uterus in this region. There
21   is no free fluid in the cul-de-sac. Comparison with prior studies
22   indicates that there has been enlargement of these myomata since
23   prior examination.

24   IMPRESSION: Live twin intrauterine gestations, approximately
25   8 weeks and 1 day maturity with a 5-day variability.

26   Three uterine myomata; two within the lower segment, and
27   the largest extending anteriorly from the lower body of the uterus.

28   _____
29   Edward Burns, MD

30   EB/urs

31   d: 6/21/—
32   t: 6/21/—   Word Count 268
33   ▪▪   SPFEMTA.3

sclerotherapy	Injection of sclerosing (causing or developing sclerosis, a hardening of an organ or tissue) solutions in the treatment of diseases.
hepatic	Pertaining to the liver.
catheter	A tube passed through the body for evacuating fluids from or injecting fluids into body cavities.

TERMINATION OF HEPATIC CYST **SCLEROTHERAPY**

1   PATIENT: Fred Grauer

2   Given that the drainage of the **hepatic** cyst has
3   decreased to near negligible levels with less than 5 cc
4   drainage per day, it was elected to terminate the
5   hepatic cyst sclerotherapy.

6   The **catheter** was removed, and a bandage placed over the
7   puncture site. The patient tolerated the procedure
8   well and left the department in good condition. He was
9   given instructions to notify the department if any
10   problems should arise.

11   IMPRESSION: Termination of hepatic cyst sclerotherapy.

12

13   Robert Matting, MD

14   RM/urs

15   d: 4/14/—
16   t: 4/14/—   Word Count 105
17   SPGASFG.7

CT	Computerized tomography.
contiguous	Being in actual contact; touching along a boundary or at a point.
transaxial	Directed at right angles to the long axis of the body or a part.
pubic symphysis	Pertaining to the junction of the pubic bones on midline in front; the bony eminence under the pubic hair.
intravenous	Within a vein.
pneumothorax	Accumulation of air or gas in the pleural cavity, resulting in collapse of the lung on the affected side.
hemothorax	Collection of blood in the pleural cavity.
hepatic laceration	A tear of the liver.
subcapsular	Below any capsule, or a capsular ligament.
hemidiaphragm	Half of the diaphragm.
splenic	Pertaining to the spleen.
perisplenic	Around the spleen.
ascites	Abnormal accumulation of serous fluid within the peritoneal cavity.
hematoma	A localized collection of extravasated blood, usually clotted, in an organ, space, or tissue.
excrete	To throw off or eliminate, as waste matter, by a normal discharge.
retroperitoneum	The space behind the peritoneum (the serous membrane reflected over the viscera and lining the abdominal cavity).
extravasation	A discharge or escape, as of blood, from a vessel into the tissues.
renal	Pertaining to the kidney.
perinephric	Around the kidney.
mesenteric	Pertaining to the mesentery (a membranous fold attaching various organs to the body wall).
transverse	Extending from side to side.
fracture	The breaking of a part, especially a bone.
distal	Farthest from the center, from a medial line, or from the trunk.

CT OF THE ABDOMEN AND PELVIS

PATIENT: Mark Smith

Contiguous 10 mm **transaxial** images were obtained from the lung bases to the **pubic symphysis** following administration of both oral and **intravenous** contrast.

There is no **pneumothorax** or **hemothorax** at the lung bases.

There is no **hepatic laceration** or **subcapsular** collection below the **hemidiaphragm**. There is no **splenic** laceration or **perisplenic** fluid collection. There is no **ascites**. There is no gastric wall **hematoma**.

Both kidneys **excrete** contrast in the **retroperitoneum**. There is no **extravasation** beyond the **renal** collecting systems. There is no subcapsular or **perinephric** fluid collection. There is no retroperitoneal hematoma. The pancreas and adrenal glands are normal.

There is no **mesenteric** hematoma. The anterior abdominal wall is intact.

The bladder is intact in the pelvis. There is no free fluid in the pelvis. There is a complete **transverse fracture** of the midshaft of the left femur with overriding of the **distal** fractured fragment.

IMPRESSION:
1. No evidence of solid organ injury.

2. Complete transverse fracture of midshaft of the left femur with overriding of the distal fractured fragment.

_____

Nicolas Caputo, MD

NC/urs

d: 12/6/—
t: 12/6/—

Word Count 205
SPGASMS.8

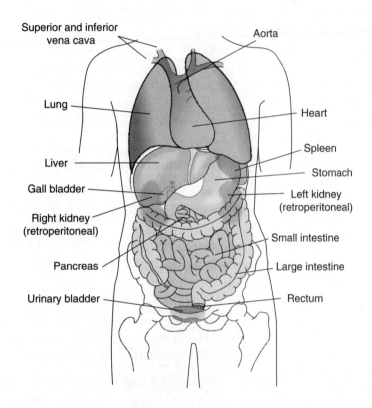

Thoracic and abdominal organs

Superior and inferior vena cava

Aorta

Lung

Heart

Spleen

Liver

Stomach

Gall bladder

Left kidney (retroperitoneal)

Right kidney (retroperitoneal)

Small intestine

Pancreas

Large intestine

Urinary bladder

Rectum

contiguous	Being in actual contact.
transaxial	Directed at right angles to the long axis of the body or a part.
pubic symphysis	Pertaining to the junction of the pubic bones on midline in front; the bony eminence under the pubic hair.
pneumothorax	A collection of air or gas in the pleural cavity. The gas enters as the result of a perforation through the chest wall or the pleura covering the lung.
hemothorax	Bloody fluid in the pleural cavity caused by the rupture of small blood vessels, due to inflammation of the lungs in pneumonia and pulmonary tuberculosis or to a malignant growth.
pleural	Pertaining to the pleura (serous membrane that enfolds both lungs).
hemidiaphragm	Half of the diaphragm.
hepatic	Pertaining to the liver.
subcapsular	Below any capsule, or a capsular ligament.
splenic	Pertaining to the spleen.
perisplenic	Around the spleen.
ascites	Abnormal accumulation of serous (producing or containing serum or a serumlike substance) fluid within the peritoneal cavity.
hematoma	A localized collection of extravasated blood, usually clotted, in an organ, space, or tissue.
retroperitoneum	The space behind the peritoneum.
cyst	A closed epithelium-lined sac or capsule containing a liquid or semisolid substance.
extravasation	A discharge or escape, as of blood, from a vessel into the tissues.
perinephric	Around the kidney.

CT OF THE ABDOMEN AND PELVIS

1   PATIENT: Sakura Nwoke

2   **Contiguous** 10 mm **transaxial** images were obtained from
3   the lung bases to the **pubic symphysis** following
4   administration of both oral and intravenous contrast.
5   There is no **pneumothorax** or **hemothorax** at the lung
6   bases. There is **bilateral pleural** reaction.

7   Below the **hemidiaphragm**, there is no **hepatic** laceration
8   or **subcapsular** collection. However, there is fatty
9   infiltration.

10   There is no **splenic** laceration or **perisplenic** fluid
11   collection. There is no **ascites**. There is no gastric
12   wall **hematoma**.

13   .In the **retroperitoneum**, there is a renal cyst arising
14   off the lower pole of the left kidney. There is also a
15   small midpole right renal **cyst**. There is no
16   **extravasation** beyond the renal collecting systems.

17   There is no subcapsular or **perinephric** fluid
18   collection. There is no retroperitoneal hematoma.
19   The pancreas and adrenal glands are normal.

20   There is no mesenteric hematoma. The anterior
21   abdominal wall is intact.

22   In the pelvis, the bladder is intact. There is no free
23   fluid in the pelvis.

24   IMPRESSION:
25   1. Right and left renal cysts.

26   2. Fatty infiltration of the liver.

27   3. No evidence of solid organ injury.

28   _____
29   James Rajpar, MD

30   JR/urs

31   d: 12/7/—
32   t: 12/7/—   Word Count 287
33   🎙   SPGASSN.9

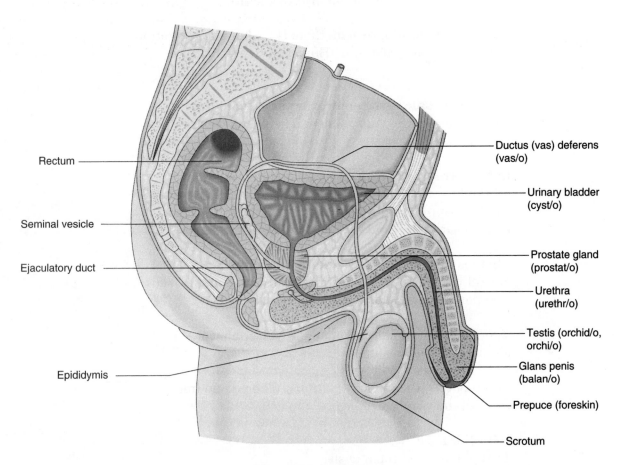

Rectum

Seminal vesicle

Ejaculatory duct

Epididymis

Ductus (vas) deferens
(vas/o)

Urinary bladder
(cyst/o)

Prostate gland
(prostat/o)

Urethra
(urethr/o)

Testis (orchid/o,
orchi/o)

Glans penis
(balan/o)

Prepuce (foreskin)

Scrotum

Male reproductive system

testis	The male gonad; either of the paired, egg-shaped glands normally situated in the scrotum.
echogenicity	Pertaining to the production or generation of reverberating sound waves as they are reflected back to their source.
hydrocele	A painless swelling of the scrotum caused by a collection of fluid in the tunica vaginalis testis, the outermost covering of the testes.
epididymis	An elongated, cordlike structure along the posterior border of the testis.

TESTICULAR ULTRASOUND

1   PATIENT: Gerald Olsen

2   The left **testis** measures 4.5 cm in length × 2.1 cm in
3   depth × 3.1 cm in transverse dimension. Normal left
4   testicular **echogenicity** is identified. There is no
5   **hydrocele** on the left side. The left **epididymis**
6   is normal.

7   _____
8   David R. Waters, MD

9   DRW/urs

10   d: 8/4/—
11   t: 8/4/—   Word Count 66
12   ▰   SPGENGO.1

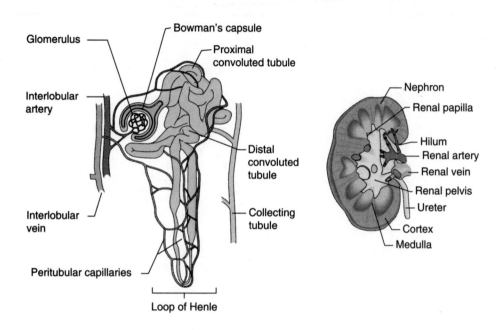

Nephron; cross section of kidney

| phleboliths | Venous calculi or concretions. |
| pelvicalyceal | Pertaining to the renal pelvis and calyx. |

PUNCTUATION REFERENCES

Line 6	comma—introductory, Rule 7
Lines 7, 8	commas—series, Rule 1
Line 11	colon—introduces information to follow, Rule 1

INTRAVENOUS UROGRAM

1   PATIENT: Clifford Barton

2   Initial film of the abdomen shows multiple pelvic
3   **phleboliths**. None of the pelvic calcifications are
4   within the urinary tract.

5   Following the injection of intravenous contrast
6   material, both kidneys are demonstrated to be smooth
7   in contour, normal in size, shape, and axis. Both
8   **pelvicalyceal** systems, ureters, and the bladder are
9   unremarkable. The bladder demonstrates excellent
10   emptying on the post void view.

11   IMPRESSION: No abnormality demonstrated.

12   _____
13   Howard Chaplin, MD

14   HC/urs

15   d: 4/15/—
16   t: 4/15/—   Word Count 77
17   �   SPGENCB.2

periphery	Outer part or surface of a body; the part away from the center.
hypoechoic	In ultrasonography, giving off few echoes.

TRANSRECTAL PROSTATIC ULTRASOUND

1   PATIENT: Harry Cohen

2   Using real-time examination, the prostate gland was
3   examined with ultrasound. The gland measures 5.9 cm in
4   length × 3.1 cm in depth × 4.9 cm in transverse
5   dimension. Prostatic volume is approximately 26 grams.

6   The gland is generally heterogeneous. In the **periphery**
7   of the left lobe, there is a **hypoechoic** nodule
8   measuring 1.7 × 0.9 × 1.4 cm. This nodule is
9   hypoechoic and partly solid. There appears to be a
10   larger hypoechoic solid nodule to the right of midline,
11   measuring approximately 2 cm in diameter. No other
12   focal nodule is identified.

13   IMPRESSION:
14   1. Small nodule left lobe peripherally.

15   2. Suspected large nodule right lobe medially.

16   3. Biopsy advised.

17   _____

18   George Dawson, MD

19   GD/urs

20   t: 6/16/—
21   d: 6/16/—   Word Count 124
22   ▣   SPGENHC.3

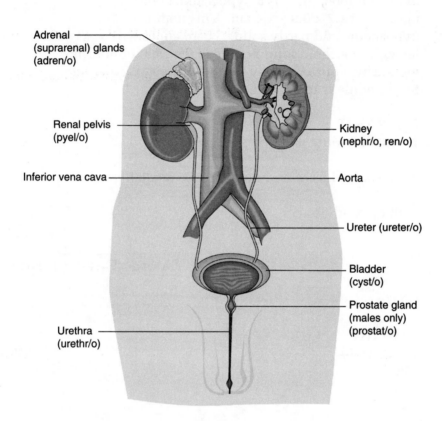

Adrenal (suprarenal) glands (adren/o)

Renal pelvis (pyel/o)

Inferior vena cava

Urethra (urethr/o)

Kidney (nephr/o, ren/o)

Aorta

Ureter (ureter/o)

Bladder (cyst/o)

Prostate gland (males only) (prostat/o)

Urinary system

renal	Pertaining to the kidney.
tomograms	Images of a tissue plane or slice produced by tomography.
calculi	Stones, usually composed of mineral salts.
pelvicalyceal	Pertaining to the renal pelvis and calyx.
UP	Ureteropelvic.
pyelolithotomy	Incision of the renal pelvis for removal of calculi.
hydronephrosis	Distention of the renal pelvis and calyces with urine.
hydroureter	Distention of the ureter with fluid, due to obstruction.

INTRAVENOUS UROGRAM

PATIENT: Danielle Caputo

Initial film of the abdomen and **renal** area **tomograms**
demonstrate no urinary tract **calculi.**

Following the injection of intravenous contrast
material, both kidneys are demonstrated to be smooth in
contour, normal in size, shape, and axis.

The right **pelvicalyceal** system and ureter are
unremarkable. The left **UP** junction shows a smooth area
of narrowing, and the patient gives a history of left
pyelolithotomy in the past. This slight narrowing is
not causing any obstruction above that level. The
remainder of the left ureter is unremarkable. No
hydronephrosis or **hydroureter** is seen on either side.

The bladder is unremarkable. A very small postvoid
residual is identified in the bladder.

IMPRESSION: No urinary tract calculi. No urinary tract
obstruction. Slight narrowing at the left UP junction which
is compatible with prior surgery in this area.

_____

James Rajpar, MD

JR/urs

d: 6/16/—
t: 6/16/—

Word Count 155
SPGENDC.4

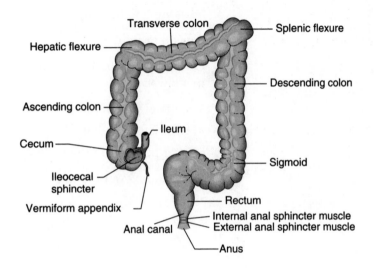

Large intestine

^{99m}Tc	Technetium 99m [a radioactive technetium] (chemistry and radiology).
tracer	A radioactive isotope capable of being incorporated into compounds, that when introduced into the body "tags" a specific molecule so that its course may be traced.
proximal	Nearest to a point of reference, as to a center or median line or to the point of attachment or origin.
transverse	Extending from side to side.
colon	The part of the large intestine extending from the cecum to the rectum.
splenic	Pertaining to the spleen.
flexure	A bend or fold.
descending	Passing from a higher place or level to a lower one.
sigmoid colon	The distal part of the colon from the level of the iliac crest to the rectum.
diverticula	Sacs or pouches in the walls of the colon.
colonoscopy	Endoscopic examination of the colon.

RADIONUCLIDE GI BLEEDING DETECTION STUDY WITH ^{99m}Tc IN VIVO TAGGING WITH RED BLOOD CELLS (20 mCi)

1   PATIENT: Tom Clarke

2   Dynamic vascular perfusion study and subsequent serial
3   images of the abdominal area show continuous
4   accumulation of **tracer** activity in the rectal region
5   indicative of active bleeding. There are multiple foci
6   of abnormal increased tracer activity in the **proximal**
7   **transverse colon**, **splenic flexure**, **descending** and
8   **sigmoid colon**. The finding could be due to different
9   foci of active bleeding probably due to rupture of
10   **diverticula**. **Colonoscopy** correlation is recommended.

11   IMPRESSION: Active bleeding from the colon. Colonoscopy
12   correlation is recommended.

13   _____
14   Catherine E. Murphy, MD

15   CEM/urs

16   d: 9/3/—
17   t: 9/3/—   Word Count 96
18   🔳   SPHEMTC.1

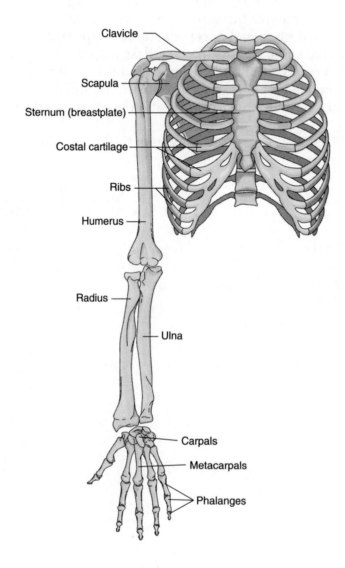

Bones of the upper extremity

SPMUSSB.1	Sally Blumberg	Terminology Preview
cortex		The outer layer of an organ or other structure, as distinguished from its inner substance.
phalanges		Bones of a finger or toe.
metacarpal		Pertaining to the bones of the metacarpus, or bones of the hand.
distal		Remote.
ulna		The inner and larger bone of the forearm, on the side opposite the thumb.
styloid		Long and pointed, like a pen or stylus.

CAT OF RIGHT HAND

1   PATIENT: Sally Blumberg

2   Multiple views of the right hand show the **cortex** of
3   the **phalanges** and **metacarpal** bones are intact. The
4   joints are unremarkable. No bony destruction or
5   fracture is seen.

6   Smooth oval density about 1 cm in diameter is seen
7   adjacent to the **distal** end of the **ulna**, most probably
8   an old fracture of the **styloid**.

9
10   John Napoli, MD

11   JN/urs

12   d: 6/10/—
13   t: 6/10/—   Word Count 81
14   ▣   SPMUSSB.1

tesla	A measure of magnetic strength.
axial	Pertaining to a line running in the main axis of the body or part of it (i.e., the axial line of the hand runs through the middle digit).
coronal	Pertaining to a corona (a coronal plane divides the body into front and back portions).
sagittal	Pertaining to a sagittal direction (a sagittal plane is a vertical plane through the longitudinal trunk dividing the body into two portions).
radiocarpal	Pertaining to the radius and carpus.
flexor retinaculum	The fascial (pertaining to or the nature of fascia—a fibrous membrane covering, supporting, and separating muscles; it also unites the skin with underlying tissue) band that holds down the flexor digits.
radioulnar	Pertaining to the radius and ulna.
carpal tunnel syndrome	A symptom complex resulting from compression of the median nerve in the carpal tunnel, with pain or tingling paresthesia (a sensation of numbness, prickling, or tingling; heightened sensitivity) in the fingers and hand, sometimes extending to the elbow.

MRI OF THE RIGHT WRIST

1   PATIENT: Violet Dong

2   MRI of the *right* wrist was performed at 1.0 **tesla**
3   utilizing **axial** and **coronal** T1 proton density and T2
4   weighted images, as well as **sagittal** T1 weighted images.

5   There is an increased T2 signal of the median nerve
6   starting at the level of the **radiocarpal** joint and
7   extending into the carpal tunnel. There is prominence
8   of the **flexor retinaculum**, and the nerve appears to be
9   compressed in a **radioulnar** dimension within the tunnel
10   itself. The adjacent flexor tendons are normal in
11   appearance. There is no significant joint effusion.

12   No marrow signal abnormality is identified, and the
13   adjacent soft tissues are unremarkable.

14   IMPRESSION: MRI findings consistent with **carpal**
15   **tunnel syndrome** of the right wrist.

16   _____
17   Charles Ferritto, MD

18   CF/urs

19   d: 6/14/—
20   t: 6/14/—   Word Count 138
21   �   SPMUSVD.3

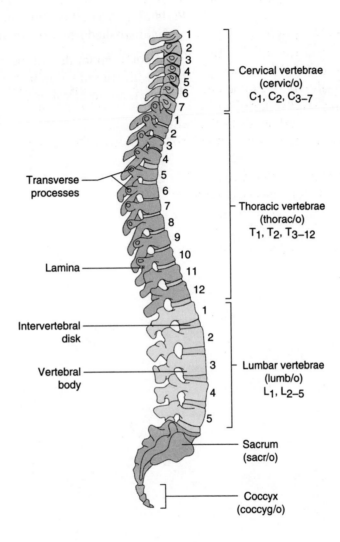

1
2
3
4
5
6
7

Cervical vertebrae
(cervic/o)
C_1, C_2, C_{3-7}

1
2
3
4
5
6
7
8
9
10
11
12

Transverse
processes

Lamina

Thoracic vertebrae
(thorac/o)
T_1, T_2, T_{3-12}

1
2
3
4
5

Intervertebral
disk

Vertebral
body

Lumbar vertebrae
(lumb/o)
L_1, L_{2-5}

Sacrum
(sacr/o)

Coccyx
(coccyg/o)

Spinal column

transverse	Extending from side to side.
trabecular	Concerning a trabecula (fibrous cord of connective tissue that serves as supporting fiber by forming a septum that extends into an organ from its wall or capsule).
cortical	Pertaining to a cortex (outer layer of an organ as distinguished from the inner medulla [marrow]).
osteoporosis	A general term for describing any disease process that results in reduction in the mass of bone per unit of volume.

QUANTITATIVE COMPUTER TOMOGRAPHY
FOR BONE MINERAL DENSITY

1   PATIENT: Ann Morgan

2   A single **transverse** section was performed through the
3   central axis of L1–L4 inclusive. Utilizing a Seimen's
4   software package, bone mineral density measurements
5   were made (mg CA-HA/mi) of **trabecular** and **cortical**
6   bone. The average value for trabecular bone
7   determination was 74.5 with a standard deviation of
8   +/– 3.4 and 195.1 for cortical bone with a standard
9   deviation of +/– 41.0.

10   The patient's calculated value was plotted on a graph
11   of age versus bone mineral density and was determined
12   to be 1.1 standard deviation below the mean.

13   IMPRESSION: Presumptive evidence of **osteoporosis**.

14   _____
15   David Dragutsky, MD

16   DD/urs

17   d: 6/13/–
18   t: 6/13/–   Word Count 118
19   SPMUSAM.4

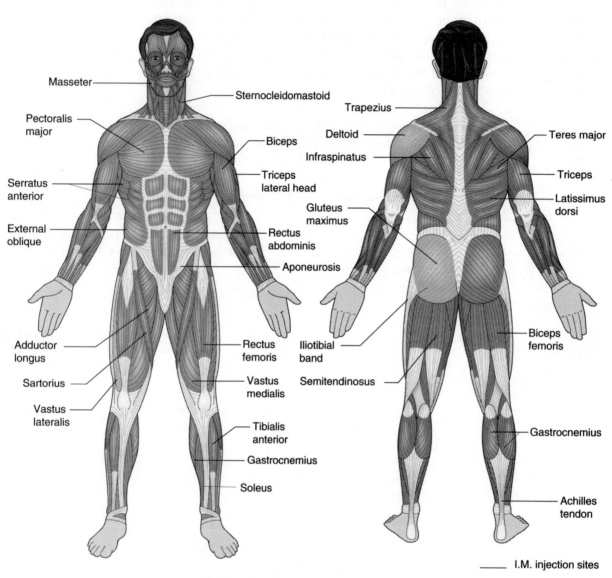

Anterior and posterior views of the muscles

Masseter

Sternocleidomastoid

Pectoralis major

Biceps

Serratus anterior

Triceps lateral head

External oblique

Rectus abdominis

Aponeurosis

Adductor longus

Rectus femoris

Sartorius

Vastus medialis

Vastus lateralis

Tibialis anterior

Gastrocnemius

Soleus

Trapezius

Deltoid

Teres major

Infraspinatus

Triceps

Latissimus dorsi

Gluteus maximus

Iliotibial band

Biceps femoris

Semitendinosus

Gastrocnemius

Achilles tendon

_____ I.M. injection sites

paracoronal	Pertaining to a coronal plane dividing the body into front and back portions.
spin echo	Spinal echoencephalogram.
cartilage	A specialized, fibrous connective tissue present in adults, and forming most of the temporary skeleton in the embryo.
diffuse	Scattered.
supraspinous	Above the spine of the scapula (shoulder blade).
infraspinous	Below the spine of the scapula.
subscapularis	Below the scapula.
glenohumeral	Pertaining to the humerus and glenoid cavity.
acromioclavicular joint	An arthrodial (pertaining to a type of synovial joint that permits only simple gliding movement within narrow limits imposed by ligaments) joint between the acromion and the acromial end of the clavicle.
hypertrophy	Increase in size of organ or structure that does not involve tumor formation.
intraosseous	Within the bone substance.
glenoid labrum	Pertaining to the liplike fibrous tissue around the margin of the glenoid socket.
subacromial	Below the acromion (lateral projection of the spine of the scapula that forms the point of the shoulder and articulates with the clavicle).
biceps	A muscle having two heads.
articular	Pertaining to a joint.
tendinitis	Inflammation of tendons and of tendon-muscle attachments.

PUNCTUATION REFERENCES

Line 17	commas—introductory, Rule 7
Line 21	period—(inside quotation marks)

MRI OF THE RIGHT SHOULDER

1   PATIENT: Robert Gatti

2   Multiple T1 proton density and T2 weighted **paracoronal**
3   images of the right shoulder were obtained utilizing
4   **spin echo** technique followed by T2 weighted gradient
5   echo axial **cartilage** sensitive sequences.

6   There is **diffuse** enlargement and intermediate signal
7   intensity within the **supraspinous** and most likely
8   **infraspinous** tendon on the T1 and proton density
9   sequence. The **subscapularis** muscle and tendon are
10   normal. No significant **glenohumeral** joint or bursal
11   effusion is seen. There is right **acromioclavicular**
12   **joint hypertrophy** extending superiorly. No
13   **intraosseous** abnormalities are seen. The **glenoid**
14   **labrum** is intact. There is perhaps minimal **subacromial**
15   fluid. The **biceps** tendon is normal. **Articular**
16   cartilage is maintained.

17   IMPRESSION: Findings, as above, most consistent with
18   **tendinitis** predominantly involving the supraspinous
19   tendon and most likely also involving the infraspinous.
20   Minimal subacromial fluid. Right acromioclavicular joint
21   hypertrophy superiorly. No definite "impingement."
22   No definite frank rotator cuff tear.

23   _____
24   Frank Mossen, MD

25   FM/urs

26   d: 4/12/—
27   t: 4/12/—   Word Count 174
28   �ци   SPMUSRG.7

proximal	Nearest to a point of reference, or to the point of attachment.
phalanges	Bones of a finger or toe.
dorsal	Directed toward or situated on the back surface.
lesion	Circumscribed area of pathologically altered tissue.
superficial	Confined to the surface.
interosseous	Situated or occurring between bones, as muscles, ligaments, or vessels; specific muscles of the hand and feet.
subcutaneous	Beneath the layers of the skin.
thenar	Fleshy eminence at base of the thumb.
extensor tendon	A cord or band of strong white fibrous tissue that connects the muscle for extension to the bone.
contiguity	Touching or in close association.
ganglion cyst	A closed epithelium-lined sac containing a liquid or semisolid substance, knotlike in appearance.
morphology	The science of the form and structure of organisms without regard to function.
musculature	The muscular system of the body, or the muscles of a particular region.

MRI OF THE RIGHT HAND

1   PATIENT: Daniel Ferber

2   An MRI of the right hand was performed at 1.0 tesla
3   utilizing axial and coronal T1 proton density and T2
4   weighted images, as well as sagittal T1 weighted images.

5   There is a 15×8 mm well-defined area of decreased T1
6   and increased T2 signal between the second and third
7   **proximal phalanges** in the **dorsal** aspect of the hand.

8   The **lesion** is immediately **superficial** to the
9   **interosseous** muscle and extends to the **subcutaneous**
10   soft tissues. The **thenar** aspect is quite round, and
11   there is a smoothly tapered narrowing of the lesion as
12   it extends across the dorsal surface of the third
13   proximal phalanx immediately deep to the **extensor**
14   **tendon**. This appearance implies **contiguity** with the
15   tendon sheath, and a **ganglion cyst** is the most likely
16   diagnosis. The tendon itself is normal in signal and
17   **morphology**.

18   The adjacent **musculature** and bony signal are normal as
19   well. No other abnormality is identified.

20   IMPRESSION: MRI findings consistent with a 15×8 mm
21   ganglion cyst in the superficial dorsal soft tissues between
22   the second and third proximal phalanges.

23

24   Reinhard Feirebend, MD

25   RF/urs

26   d: 4/12/—
27   t: 4/12/—   Word Count 210
28   SPMUSDF.9

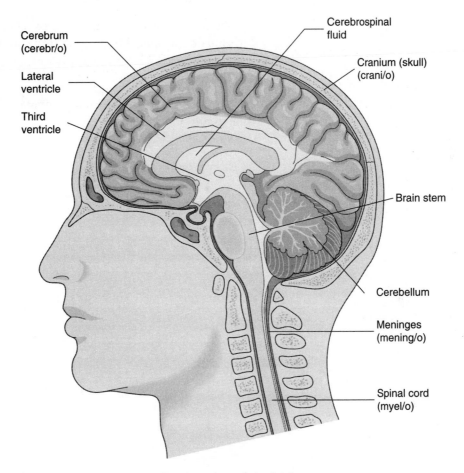

Cerebrum
(cerebr/o)

Lateral
ventricle

Third
ventricle

Cerebrospinal
fluid

Cranium (skull)
(crani/o)

Brain stem

Cerebellum

Meninges
(mening/o)

Spinal cord
(myel/o)

Cross section of the brain

contiguous	Being in actual contact.
ventricles	Small cavities or chambers, as in the brain or heart.
dilatation	The condition of being dilated or stretched beyond normal dimensions.
parenchyma	The essential or functional elements of an organ.
intracranial	Within the cranium.
infarcts	Localized areas of ischemic necrosis (a type of tissue death caused by coagulation) produced by occlusion of the arterial supply or the venous drainage of the parts.
atrophy	Decrease in size of a normally developed organ or tissue.

CT HEAD

1   PATIENT: Kathy Cruz

2   CLINICAL HISTORY: Change in mental status.

3   **Contiguous** 10 mm axial images of the brain were
4   obtained without the use of contrast.

5   The **ventricles** are midline and without evidence of
6   **dilatation** or mass effect. No extra-axial fluid
7   collection is seen. The brain **parenchyma** does not
8   demonstrate any evidence of an **intracranial** hemorrhage.

9   No **infarcts** are seen. There is generalized cerebral
10   **atrophy** noted which is consistent with the patient's
11   HIV status. No other abnormalities are seen.

12   IMPRESSION:
13   1. Generalized cerebral atrophy.

14   2. No evidence of acute brain pathology.

15   _____
16   Claire A. Molloy, MD

17   CAM/urs

18   d: 9/8/—
19   t: 9/8/—   Word Count 98
20   SPNERKC.1

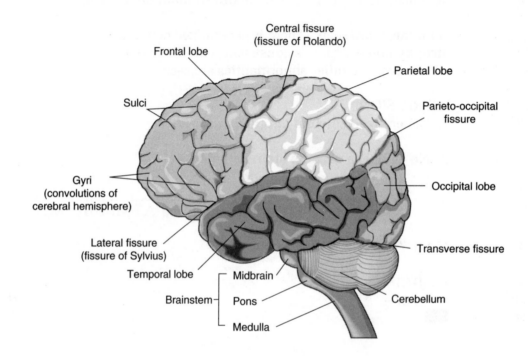

Lateral view of the brain

SPNERFG.2	Felix Greene	Terminology Preview
MRI		Magnetic resonance imaging.
sagittal		Pertaining to a sagittal direction (a sagittal plane is a vertical plane through the longitudinal trunk dividing the body into two portions).
axial		Pertaining to an axis; a real or imaginary line that runs through the center of a body, or about which a part revolves.
proton		An elementary particle of mass number 1, with a positive charge equal to the negative charge of the electron.
density		The degree of blackness on a radiograph.
angiography		Radiography of vessels of the body.
intracranial vasculature		The vascular system within the cranium.
adjuvant		Assisting or aiding.
ventricular dilatation		Pertaining to the expansion or stretching of a ventricle (one of the cavities of the brain).
cortical sulci		In anatomy, a general term for a depression, especially one on the brain surface.
vascular		Pertaining to blood vessels or indicative of a copious blood supply.
aneurysm		A sac formed by the localized dilatation of the wall of an artery, vein, or the heart.
anomaly		Marked deviation from normal.
atrophy		Decrease in size of a normally developed organ or tissue; wasting.

MRI OF THE BRAIN

1   PATIENT: Felix Greene

2   An MRI of the brain was performed on a 1.0 tesla magnet
3   utilizing selected **sagittal** T1, **axial** T1 **proton density**
4   and T2 weighted images. MRI **angiography** of the
5   **intracranial vasculature** was performed as an **adjuvant**
6   sequence.

7   There is moderate **ventricular dilatation** associated
8   with prominence of the **cortical sulci**. There is no
9   mass effect. No dominant signal abnormality is
10   identified in the brain. There is no extra-axial
11   collection, and the **vascular** flow voids are maintained.

12 . MRI angiography demonstrates no evidence of
13   intracranial **aneurysm** or vascular **anomaly**.

14   IMPRESSION: Age appropriate cerebral **atrophy**.

15   _____
16   Jonathan Hess, MD

17   JH/urs

18   d: 4/13/—
19   t: 4/13/—   Word Count 121
20   ▄▄   SPNERFG.2

MRI		Magnetic resonance imaging.
thoracic spine		That part of the spinal column between the cervical and lumbar curves containing 12 vertebrae.
sagittal		Pertaining to a sagittal direction (a sagittal plane is a vertical plane through the longitudinal trunk dividing the body into two portions).
axial		Pertaining to a line running in the main axis of the body or part of it.
vertebral		Pertaining to a vertebra.
intradural		Within or beneath the dura mater.
posterior		Directed toward or situated at the back; opposite of anterior.
ventral subarachnoid		Pertaining to the anterior or front side of the space between the arachnoid and the pia mater.
paraspinal		Near the spine.
intrinsic		Situated entirely within or pertaining exclusively to a part.

MRI OF THORACIC SPINE

1   PATIENT: Donald Ercolano

2   MRI of the thoracic spine was performed at 1.0 tesla
3   utilizing **sagittal** T1 proton density and T2 weighted
4   images, as well as **axial** T1 weighted images.

5   The **vertebral** bodies are of normal height, signal
6   intensity, and alignment. The thoracic cord is normal
7   in contour and signal intensity. No **intradural** mass is
8   identified.

9   At T2–T3 there is a small **posterior** ridge on the
10   right which results in a mild mass effect upon the
11   **ventral subarachnoid** space without cord compression.

12   The remaining disk levels are unremarkable. The
13   **paraspinal** soft tissues are normal.

14   IMPRESSION:
15   1. No **intrinsic** cord lesion.

16   2. Small posterior ridge at T2–T3 on the right.

17   _____
18   Shankar P. Iyer, MD

19   SPI/urs

20   d: 4/12/–
21   t: 4/12/–   Word Count 139
22   ▄▄   SPNERDE.3

SPNERJM.4	Jennifer Martin	Terminology Preview
cervical spine		The upper portion of the spinal column containing seven cervical bones (neck).
axial		Pertaining to a line running in the main axis of the body or part of it.
sagittal		Pertaining to a sagittal direction (a sagittal plane is a vertical plane through the longitudinal trunk dividing the body into two portions).
spin echo		Spinal echoencephalogram.
protrusion		Extension beyond the usual limits, or above a plane surface.
encroachment		Situated outside the usual or proper limits.
intradural		Within or beneath the dura mater (a fibrous connective tissue membrane, the outermost of the meninges covering the spinal cord and brain).
paraspinal		Near the spine.
craniocervical		Relating to the skull and cervical spine.
facet		A small, smooth area on a bone.
herniation		Abnormal protrusion of an organ or other body structure.

PUNCTUATION REFERENCES

Line 9	comma—series, Rule 1
Line 9	hyphens—range of numbers
Line 10	comma—two-adjective modifier, Rule 2
Line 10	hyphen—range of numbers
Line 11	commas—series, Rule 1
Line 16	hyphen—range of numbers
Line 18	hyphen—range of numbers

MRI OF THE **CERVICAL SPINE**

1   PATIENT: Jennifer Martin

2   Multiple T1 weighted **axial** and **sagittal** images of the
3   cervical spine were obtained utilizing **spin echo**
4   technique followed by T2 weighted gradient echo
5   sagittal sequences.

6   There is moderate central C5–6 disk **protrusion** with
7   accompanying **encroachment**. There is minimal loss of
8   disk height but preservation of signal at this level.

9   The C2–3, 3–4, 6–7, and C7–T1 disk levels are normal.

10   There is perhaps a subtle, central C4–5 disk bulge.

11   Vertebral height, alignment, and marrow signal are
12   maintained. No **intradural** or **paraspinal** abnormalities
13   are seen. The cervical cord and **craniocervical**
14   junction are normal. No significant degenerative **facet**
15   disease is present.

16   IMPRESSION: Moderate central C5–6 disk **herniation**.

17   No significant cervical cord or nerve root involvement.

18   Minimal central C4–5 disk bulge.

19   _____
20   James Barton, MD

21   JB/urs

22   d: 4/13/–
23   t: 4/13/–   Word Count 151
24   �   SPNERJM.4

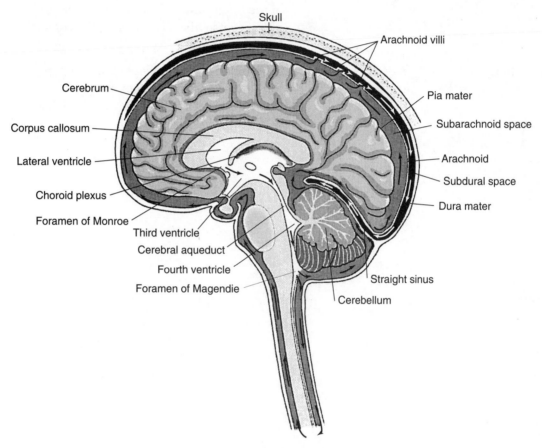

Cross section of the brain

gadolinium	A chemical element, atomic number 64, atomic weight 157.25.
intraparenchymal	Within the essential parts of an organ that are concerned with its function in contradistinction to its framework.
brain stem	The stemlike portion of the brain connecting the cerebral hemispheres with the spinal cord.
corpus callosum	An arched mass of white matter in the depths of the longitudinal fissure, and made up of transverse fibers connecting the cerebral hemispheres.
cerebellum	The part of the metencephalon (the part of the central nervous system comprising the pons and cerebellum) situated on the back of the brain stem.

MRI OF THE BRAIN
WITH ATTENTION TO THE INTERNAL AUDITORY CANALS

1   PATIENT: Peter Smyth

2   Multiple thin section T1 weighted axial images were
3   obtained through the seventh to eighth nerve complexes.

4   Proton density and T2 weighted axial images of the
5   brain were obtained. Spin echo technique was utilized.

6   T1 weighted sagittal images are available.

7   Please note the patient could not tolerate **gadolinium**
8   due to nausea prior to injection.

9   The seventh to eighth nerve complexes are well visualized
10   and demonstrate normal signal intensity and contour.
11   No focal **intraparenchymal** or extra-axial abnormality
12   is seen. The ventricles and subarachnoid spaces retain
13   their normal configuration. The **brain stem**, **corpus**
14   **callosum,** and **cerebellum** are normal. Normal
15   intracranial vascular flow void is maintained. The
16   orbital contents are normal. Normal signal void is
17   seen within the paranasal sinuses.

18   IMPRESSION: Normal MRI of the brain with attention
19   to the internal auditory canal despite lack of gadolinium.

20   _____

21   Vincent Verdi, MD

22   VV/urs

23   d: 6/16/—
24   t: 6/16/—   Word Count 164
25   ▄▄   SPNERPS.5

lumbar spine		The lower part of the spinal column between the thorax and the pelvis containing five vertebrae.
conus		Conical (conelike) portion of the lower spine.
intradural		Within or beneath the dura mater (outer membrane covering the spinal cord and brain).
thecal		Pertaining to the theca (a sheath of investing membrane).
congenital		Existing from the time of birth.
foramenal		Pertaining to the spinous foramen (opening in the spine of the sphenoid bone through which passes the middle meningeal artery).
stenosis		Narrowing or contraction of a body passage or opening.

MRI OF **LUMBAR SPINE**

1   PATIENT: Anthony Ferrara

2   An MRI of the lumbar spine was performed on a 1.0 tesla
3   magnet utilizing sagittal T1 proton density and T2
4   weighted images, as well as axial proton density
5   weighted images.

6   The vertebral bodies are of normal height, signal
7   intensity, and alignment. The **conus** is normal in
8   position, and there is no **intradural** abnormality.

9   There is a loss of T2 signal at the L4–L5 disk space.

10   The disk itself is diffusely bulging, resulting in a
11   mass effect upon the ventral aspect of the **thecal** sac.

12   This is somewhat more prominent due to mild **congenital**
13   narrowing of the canal at this level.

14   There is a mild diffuse disk bulge at L3–L4 with no
15   evidence of spinal or **foramenal** compromise. The
16   remaining disk levels are unremarkable.

17   IMPRESSION: Mild spinal **stenosis** at L4–L5 due to a
18   diffuse disk bulge with mild congenital narrowing
19   of the canal.

20   _____
21   Ronald Segrems, MD

22   RS/urs

23   d: 6/16/–
24   t: 6/16/–   Word Count 169
25   ▭   SPNERAF.6

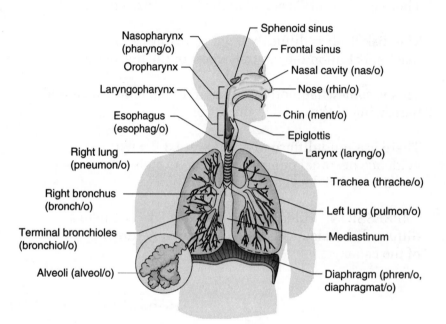

Respiratory system

infrahilar	Beneath the root of the lungs at the level of the fourth and fifth dorsal vertebrae.
truncated	Having a square end as if it were cut off; lacking an apex.
parenchyma	The essential or functional parts of an organ as distinguished from its framework.
osseous	Bonelike.

PORTABLE FILM OF THE THORAX

1   PATIENT: Ariel Eusebio

2   The right diaphragm is elevated. The right **infrahilar**
3   space is **truncated** with crowding of the truncal markings.
4   The remainder of the pulmonary **parenchyma** is unremarkable.
5   Cardiac silhouette is enlarged in its transverse diameter.
6   The visualized **osseous** structures appear intact. Bilateral
7   cardiac monitor leads are present.

8   IMPRESSION: Elevated right diaphragm. Recommend
9   real-time abdominal sonography for further evaluation.

10 _____

11   Philip Black, MD

12 PB/urs

13 d: 6/16/—
14 t: 6/16/—   Word Count 84
15   ◼   SPRESAE.1

peribronchial	Around a bronchus or bronchi.
parenchyma	The essential or functional elements of an organ.
intramural	Within the wall of an organ.
CVP	Central venous pressure.
brachycephalic	Having a short, wide head.
supraclavicular	Above the clavicle.
endarterectomy	Excision of thickened atheromatous (fatty degeneration of the walls of the larger arteries occurring in atherosclerosis) areas of the innermost coat of an artery.
Cytoxan	Trademark for preparations of cyclophosphamide, an antineoplastic (preventing the development, growth, or proliferation of malignant cells) agent.
Oncovin	Trademark for a preparation of vincristine sulfate.
prednisone	A glucocorticoid (a general classification of adrenal cortical hormones that are primarily active in protecting against stress and in affecting protein and carbohydrate metabolism).
bleomycin	A polypeptide antibiotic mixture having antineoplastic properties, obtained from cultures of *Streptomyces verticellus.*

PORTABLE FILM OF THE THORAX

1   PATIENT: Barry Ahrens

2   Portable film of the thorax discloses several **peribronchial**
3   infiltrations, extending anteriorly from the right lung root
4   to the diaphragm. Both sides of the diaphragm are smooth
5   in contour although flattened. The remainder of the
6   pulmonary **parenchyma** is hyper-illuminated. Uncoiling
7   of the thoracic aorta is apparent with **intramural**
8   calcification of the aortic arch. Cardiac silhouette is
9   normal in its transverse diameter. A **CVP** line is present
10   in the **brachycephalic** vessel. The nasogastric tube is
11   evident with its tip in the body of the stomach.
12   Endotracheal tube is also identified with its tip on the
13   level of the superior border of D3. Metallic sutures are
14   present in the **supraclavicular** regions secondary to
15   an **endarterectomy**.

16   IMPRESSION: Right lower lobe infiltrations.

17   **Cytoxan Oncovin prednisone bleomycin** (COPB).

18   Status post current endotracheal assist.

19   _____
20   Jane Dugan, MD

21   JD/urs

22   d: 6/16/—
23   t: 6/16/—   Word Count 148
24   ▰   SPRESBA.2

Operative Reports

OVERVIEW

In this section the student will be transcribing operative reports specific to the cardiovascular, gastrointestinal, integumentary, lymphatic, musculoskeletal, and respiratory body systems.

Terminology previews are provided for each report. Punctuation references illustrating uses of the comma, hyphen, and semicolon are provided in four reports.

OPERATIVE REPORTS

Operative reports are prepared detailing each step of a patient's operation. There are several sections common to this type of report, but variations will occur depending upon the formatting preferences of the individual hospital. Most hospitals use templates (preprinted forms) containing sections to be completed with the required information.

Use of a Macro

It is recommended that the student prepare a macro on a word processor to contain the heading, OPERATIVE REPORT, and side headings for PATIENT:, DATE:, PREOPERATIVE DIAGNOSIS:, POSTOPERATIVE DIAGNOSIS:, and PROCEDURE: (as shown in the transcribed reports). The macro can be named and retrieved with "Alt o". (Consult your instructional manual for macro preparation, as needed.)

Multiple Page Headings

When the report exceeds one page, key the patient's name, and page number beginning on the first line of each succeeding page. For example,

John Higgins

Page 2

Saving and Coding Transcripts

The student should name and save each transcribed report with the code provided at the end of each report.

INSTRUCTIONAL OBJECTIVES

In this chapter, the student will:

1. Transcribe operative reports of varying lengths in report format.
2. Learn terminology relative to the cardiovascular, gastrointestinal, integumentary, lymphatic, musculoskeletal, and respiratory body systems.
3. Reinforce understanding of the use of the comma (introductory, series, conjunction, title following a person's name, two-adjective modifier, and parenthetical), hyphen (compound modifier), and semicolon (independent clauses without a conjunction).

REMINDERS: Preview highlighted medical terms and punctuation references in the report.
Listen to the tape to become familiar with it.
Transcribe the report inserting punctuation "cues."
Print out a hard copy.
Check carefully your transcribed report word by word to the text transcript.

THE TRANSCRIPT IN THE TEXT IS CHECKED <u>ONLY AFTER</u> YOU HAVE COMPLETED YOUR TRANSCRIPTION.

Record the number of lines transcribed and the number of minutes needed to complete the report.
Make corrections; submit the corrected transcript to your instructor.

OPERATIVE REPORTS INDEX

	Patient Name	Code Name	Word Count
CAR	JOHN HIGGINS	ORCARJH.1	174
	ANNA TAN	ORCARAT.2	252
	MARLENE TURRELL	ORCARMT.3*	359
	NICHOLAS VOGIATZIS	ORCARNV.4	433
	MARTINA JOHNSON	ORCARMJ.5	626
	PAUL HAYWORTH	ORCARPH.6	876
GAS	DANIELLA PESTOVA	ORGASDP.1	181
	NORMAN KEEFE	ORGASNK.2*	227
	EVA HERZIGOVA	ORGASEH.3	282
	HENRY KANTER	ORGASHK.4	322
	SALVATORE MINO	ORGASSM.5	506
INT	SHERRI SHELLOOE	ORINTSS.1	179
	SHEILA TUTTLE	ORINTST.2	229
	CONNIE SHUTE	ORINTCS.3*	232
	MICHAEL WALLACE	ORINTMW.4*	324
LYM	JONATHAN LEE	ORLYMJL.1	203
	NATALIE TUCKER	ORLYMNT.2	280
MUS	JUDITH BRYDEN	ORMUSJB.1	231
	MICHELE VALDEZ	ORMUSMV.2	259
	JOHN GIBLIN	ORMUSJG.3	348
RES	MICHAEL JULES	ORRESMJ.1	179
	PATRICK ATTARDI	ORRESPA.2	216
	DONALD BRIGGS	ORRESDB.3	304

*Punctuation References

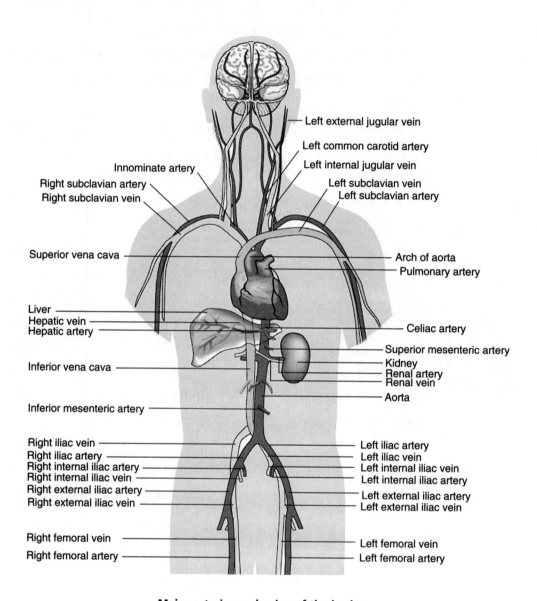

Major arteries and veins of the body

Crohn's disease	Inflammation of the intestinal tract, commonly of the terminal (end) portion of ileum.
hyperalimentation	Administration or consumption of nutrients beyond minimum normal requirements, in an attempt to replace nutritional deficiencies.
subclavian	Beneath the clavicle.
percutaneously	Process going through the skin.
IV	Intravenous (within a vein or veins).

1 PATIENT: John Higgins

2 DATE: 6/25/–

3 SURGEON: Edward J. Gordon, MD

4 PREOPERATIVE DIAGNOSIS: **Crohn's disease** requiring
5 central venous access for **hyperalimentation**.

6 POSTOPERATIVE DIAGNOSIS: Crohn's disease requiring
7 central venous access for hyperalimentation.

8 OPERATION: Insertion of left-sided **subclavian** double-
9 lumen central venous catheter.

10 ANESTHESIA: 1% lidocaine.

11 PROCEDURE: The patient was placed in the supine
12 position with the neck extended to the right side. The
13 left side of the chest was prepared and draped in the
14 usual manner using Betadine solution. The subclavian
15 vein on the left side was **percutaneously** and easily
16 entered, and the guide wire was advanced into the
17 superior vena cava. The double-lumen central venous
18 catheter with VitaCuff was placed through the guide
19 wire into the superior vena cava. Good blood flow was
20 obtained. The catheter was sutured to the skin
21 using 2-0 silk sutures and connected to **IV** solution.

22 A dry sterile dressing was applied.

23 The patient tolerated the procedure well.

24 _____
25 Edward J. Gordon, MD

26 EJG/urs

27 d: 6/25/–
28 t: 6/27/–   **Word Count 174**
29   **ORCARJH.1**

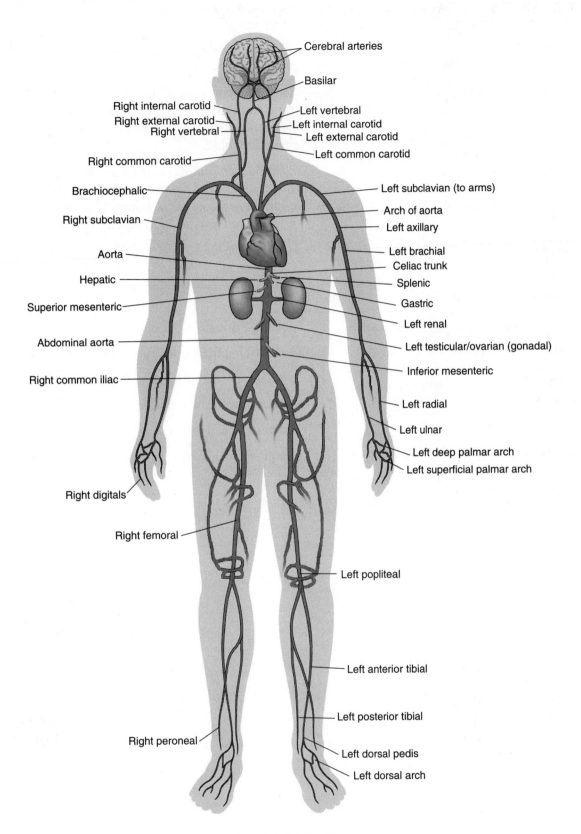

Cerebral arteries

Basilar

Right internal carotid

Right external carotid

Right vertebral

Left vertebral

Left internal carotid

Left external carotid

Right common carotid

Left common carotid

Brachiocephalic

Left subclavian (to arms)

Right subclavian

Arch of aorta

Left axillary

Aorta

Left brachial

Hepatic

Celiac trunk

Superior mesenteric

Splenic

Gastric

Left renal

Abdominal aorta

Left testicular/ovarian (gonadal)

Right common iliac

Inferior mesenteric

Left radial

Left ulnar

Left deep palmar arch

Left superficial palmar arch

Right digitals

Right femoral

Left popliteal

Left anterior tibial

Left posterior tibial

Right peroneal

Left dorsal pedis

Left dorsal arch

Arterial distribution

Acquired Immune Deficiency Syndrome	AIDS. A disease marked by a decrease in the immune response.
Hickman catheter	A central venous tube providing access for IV infusion or dialysis (the passage of a solute [substance dissolved in a solution] through a membrane).
lactated Ringer's	A sterile solution of specified amounts of calcium chloride, potassium chloride, sodium chloride, and sodium lactate in water for injection intravenously to replace electrolytes.
supine	Lying on the back.
subcutaneous	Beneath the skin.
clavicle	Collarbone.
percutaneous	Effected through the skin.
superior vena cava	Drains blood from the upper portion of the body.
fluoroscopy	Examination with a fluorescent screen.
medial	Pertaining to the middle.
caudad	In a posterior direction.
pneumothorax	The presence of air or gas in the pleural cavity.

PATIENT: Anna Tan

PREOPERATIVE DIAGNOSIS: **Acquired Immune Deficiency Syndrome.**

POSTOPERATIVE DIAGNOSIS: Acquired Immune Deficiency Syndrome.

OPERATION: Insertion of **Hickman catheter.**

ESTIMATED BLOOD LOSS: Approximately 5 cc.

IV FLUIDS: Approximately 250 cc
of **lactated Ringer's.**

ANESTHESIA: Local.

PROCEDURE: Patient was brought to the operating room
and placed in the **supine** position. The left shoulder
was prepped and draped in the usual sterile manner.
Approximately 8 cc of 1% lidocaine without epinephrine
was used to infiltrate the skin and **subcutaneous** tissue
in the area of the **clavicle.** Access was gained to the
subclavian vein via the **percutaneous** approach with good
blood return. The double-lumen Hickman catheter was fed
over a wire and introduced through the subclavian vein.
Position of the tip was confirmed to be in the **superior
vena cava** by **fluoroscopy.** A subcutaneous tunnel was
made from the percutaneous puncture site down to a
level of approximately 2 cm **medial** and 2 cm **caudad** of
the left nipple.

The Hickman catheter was then brought down the tunnel
and brought exteriorly at the level of the exit site
with good venous return from all three ports. A stat
portable chest x-ray in the recovery room revealed no
pneumothorax as well as the catheter tip being in
position in the superior vena cava. The wounds were
dressed with telfa and tegaderm in the operating room.
Patient tolerated the procedure well and went to the
recovery room in stable condition.

_____

James Lap, MD

JL/urs

d: 1/4/—
t: 1/4/—
⊟

Word Count 254
ORCARAT.2

MediPort catheter	Catheter (tube) used for insertion of medication.
neuroleptic	A narcotic analgesic (a drug to relieve pain and produce sleep).
prepped	Prepared for surgery.
draped	Covered parts of the body other than those to be examined or operated on.
subclavian	Pertaining to beneath the clavicle.
lidocaine	A local anesthetic.
epinephrine	Adrenaline. The most potent stimulant resulting in increased heart rate and force of contraction, vasoconstriction, or vasodilation (a decrease in the caliber [diameter] of blood vessels).
subcutaneous	Beneath the skin.
deltopectoral groove	A narrow, elongated depression in shoulder prominence and chest.
transverse incision	Cut crosswise.
deltoid	Triangular-shaped (deltoid muscle covers the shoulder prominence).
pectoral	Relating to the chest.
cephalic vein	Cranial vein.
venotomy	Incision into a vein for the purpose of drawing blood.
fluoroscopy	Examination of the tissues and deep structures of the body by x-ray, using the fluoroscope.
scapular	Relating to the shoulder blade.
cannulation	Insertion of a cannula tube into a cavity.
aborted	Discontinued effort or project before its completion.
incision	Cut.
inferior	Situated below or directed downward.
aspiration	Removal, by suction, of a gas or fluid from a body cavity.
atrium	A chamber or cavity to which are connected several chambers or passageways.
interrupted sutures	Sutures formed by single stitches inserted separately and fixed by tying ends together.
inflated	Distended by a fluid or gas.
pneumothorax	Collapse of the lung.
RA	Right atrium.

PUNCTUATION REFERENCES

Line 11	comma—introductory, Rule 7
Line 12	comma—conjunction, Rule 3
Line 18	comma—conjunction, Rule 3
Line 19	comma—introductory, Rule 7
Lines 21, 22	commas—parenthetical, Rule 10
Lines 23, 26	comma—conjunction, Rule 3
Line 36	hyphen—lowercase and hyphenate for noun, verb, or adjective
Lines 33, 37	comma—conjunction, Rule 3

PATIENT: Marlene Turrell

PREOPERATIVE DIAGNOSIS: Central venous access.

POSTOPERATIVE DIAGNOSIS: Central venous access.

OPERATION: Insertion of **MediPort Catheter**.

ANESTHESIA: Local **neuroleptic**.

ANESTHESIOLOGIST: Maureen LaSala, MD

PROCEDURE: The patient was **prepped** and **draped** over the right **subclavian** region using 1% **lidocaine** without **epinephrine.** Approximately 3 to 4 cc were injected into the skin and **subcutaneous** tissue in the right **deltopectoral groove**. Using a #15 blade, a 4 cm **transverse incision** was made through the skin, and the subcutaneous tissue was bluntly dissected down to locate the **deltoid** and **pectoral** muscle edges and the subsequent groove. Blunt dissection again was followed down to the **cephalic vein**. This vein was isolated using two 4-0 silks.

A **venotomy** was made using a #11 blade, and the MediPort catheter was passed through. At approximately 5 cm, there was resistance though the catheter did pass easily. **Fluoroscopy** showed that the catheter was, in fact, curling around the level of the **scapular** vein.

Cannulation of this vein was **aborted,** and a subclavian stick was performed on the right side through the **incision** already made. This procedure was achieved easily, and the MediPort catheter was inserted into the subclavian vein. The MediPort was inserted into the subcutaneous tissue **inferior** to the wound. A pocket was made using blunt dissection for that port. The port was sutured to the deep tissue using 4-0 chromics ×2 at each side. The port did have good return on **aspiration** and was flushed with some heparin solution.

The position of the port was checked with fluoroscopy, and it was found to be in good position at the level of the right **atrium**. The deep tissue was closed using 4-0 chromic **interrupted sutures**. Postop chest x-ray showed the lung to be fully **inflated** without **pneumothorax,** and

38   the catheter to be at the level of the **RA**. Dressing was
39   applied. The patient tolerated the procedure well and
40   was transferred to the recovery room.

41   ESTIMATED BLOOD LOSS: Approximately 20 to 40 cc.

42   SUTURES USED: 4-0 chromic, 5-0 silk.

43   CATHETER USED: MediPort Catheter.

44   CASE: Clean.

45   _____
46   Nicholas Pacholka, MD

47   NP/urs

48   d: 1/5/—
49   t: 1/5/—   Word Count 359
50   📼   ORCARMT.3

pericardial effusion	Fluid in the pericardial cavity, between the visceral and parietal pericardium (the middle serous layer of the pericardial sac, lining the fibrous layer).
pericarditis	Inflammation of the pericardium.
thoracotomy	Surgical incision of the chest wall.
general endotracheal	Anesthesia administered with a tube passed through the trachea.
platelets	Thrombocytes; play an important role in blood coagulation.
myocardium	The middle layer of the walls of the heart composed of heart muscle.
Betadine	Trade name for povidone-iodine, a topical anti-infective.
anteriorly	Pertaining to the front, abdominal side of the body.
scalpel	A small, straight surgical knife with a convex edge and thin, keen blade.
dermis	The skin.
electrocautery	Cauterization using electric current.
subcutaneous	Beneath the skin.
pectoralis	One of four muscles of the anterior upper portion of the chest.
intercostal	Between the ribs.
pleura	Serous membrane enfolding both lungs and reflected upon the wall of the thorax and diaphragm.
forceps	Pincers for holding, seizing, or extracting in surgery.
serous fluid	Liquid of the body that is, in part, secreted by serous membranes.
cultures	Propagation of microorganisms or of living cells in special media conducive to their growth.
hemostasis	Arrest/stop bleeding.

1   PATIENT: Nicholas Vogiatzis

2   PREOPERATIVE DIAGNOSIS: **Pericardial effusion.**

3   POSTOPERATIVE DIAGNOSIS: **Pericarditis.** Small
4   pericardial effusions.

5   OPERATION: Left **thoracotomy** and pericardial window.

6   ANESTHESIA: **General endotracheal.**

7   ESTIMATED BLOOD LOSS: 20 cc. Fluids—2 units of
8   packed red blood cells, 1000 cc of Ringer's lactate,
9   8 units of **platelets**.

10   FINDINGS: Less than 20 cc of pericardial effusions,
11   thickened pericardium, and thickened **myocardium**.

12   PROCEDURE: The patient was placed on the operating
13   room table and after the successful induction of
14   general anesthesia, the left chest was shaved and
15   prepped with **Betadine** solution in the usual sterile
16   fashion. We then draped the left chest in the usual sterile
17   fashion. We made an approximately 3-inch long
18   incision over the sixth rib **anteriorly** with a **scalpel**
19   through the **dermis** and, using **electrocautery**, went
20   through the **subcutaneous** tissue and **pectoralis** major
21   muscle to go down to the layer of the sixth rib. We
22   went over the top of the superior aspect of the
23   superior rib and dissected off the **intercostal** muscles
24   and then went into the **pleura** over the anterior aspect
25   of the superior sixth rib. After entering the pleural
26   cavity, there was a whitish tinge to the left lung. We
27   packed away the lung with a wet gauze and then observed
28   the myocardium. It was enlarged and thickened, however,
29   it did not appear to be dense with fluid. Using the
30   DeBakey **forceps**, we made an approximate 6 cm surface
31   area disk removed from the left anterior aspect of the
32   myocardium anterior to the phrenic nerve. Inside the
33   pericardium, there were less than 20 to 30 cc of **serous**
34   **fluid** which was sent for various **cultures**. After
35   removing the disk, we copiously irrigated the
36   pericardium and left chest, and the solution was taken
37   up. Using electrocautery, we cauterized the edges of
38   the pericardium. After judging that **hemostasis** was
39   adequate, we began to close the chest by first placing
40   a #36 chest tube over the ninth rib at the level of the

41 anterior iliac spine and placed with the tip of the
42 chest tube at the apex. The hole of the chest tube
43 which was enlarged inside the chest was tied with #2-0
44 silk. We reapproximated the ribs using a #2 pericostal
45 figure-of-eight chromic sutures and tied this. We then
46 reapproximated the pectoralis major with #0 Vicryl and
47 reapproximated the subcutaneous tissue with #2-0 Vicryl.
48 The skin was reapproximated with #3-0 nylon vertical
49 mattress sutures. A sterile dressing was placed over
50 this, and the patient was taken to the recovery room in
51 stable condition.

52 _____

53 Richard B. Kressel, MD

54 RBK/urs

55 d: 12/20—
56 t: 12/20/—   Word Count 433
57 ▦   ORCARNV.4

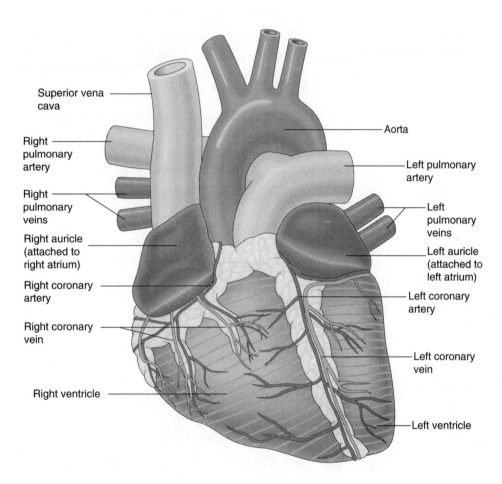

Superior vena cava

Right pulmonary artery

Right pulmonary veins

Right auricle (attached to right atrium)

Right coronary artery

Right coronary vein

Right ventricle

Aorta

Left pulmonary artery

Left pulmonary veins

Left auricle (attached to left atrium)

Left coronary artery

Left coronary vein

Left ventricle

External structure of the heart

LAD	Left anterior descending (coronary artery).
epigastric	Relating to the epigastrium (region over the pit of the stomach).
congestive heart failure	CHF; a condition in which the heart is unable to pump its required amount of blood.
hiatal hernia	Protrusion of the stomach upward into the mediastinal cavity through the esophageal hiatus of the diaphragm.
cardiac catheterization	A thin, flexible tube (catheter) is introduced into a vein or artery and is guided into the heart for purposes of detecting pressures and patterns of blood flow.
angiography	A diagnostic procedure involving injection of an x-ray dye into the bloodstream, followed by chest x-rays to show the dimensions of the heart and large blood vessels.
left ventricle dysfunction	Difficult or abnormal function of the lower chamber of the heart.
occlusion	Closure of a blood vessel.
stenosis	A narrowing of one of the cardiac valves.
ostial	Relating to any orifice; a small opening.
intravenous	Within a vein or veins.
heparin	An anticoagulant used in prevention and treatment of thrombosis and embolism.
revascularization	Reestablishment of blood supply.
supine	Lying on the back.
endotracheal	Within the trachea (windpipe).
median	Central; middle; lying in the midline.
sternotomy	Incision into or through the sternum.
saphenous	Relating to or associated with a saphenous vein; denoting a number of structures in the leg.
plasmalyte	A replenisher of plasma.
papaverine	A mild analgesic (a drug that relieves pain).
electrocautery	The process of using a metal cauterizing instrument for directing a current through a local area of tissue.
hemoclips	Metal clips used to ligate blood vessels.
pericardium	A saclike membrane surrounding the heart.

anterior	The front of the body.
cannula	A tube that can be inserted into a cavity.
distal	Away from the beginning of a structure; away from the center.
anastomoses	Openings created by surgery, trauma, or disease between two or more normally separated spaces or organs.
defibrillated	Arrested fibrillation of the cardiac muscle with restoration of the normal rhythm.
arteriotomies	Any surgical incisions into the lumen of an artery.
weaned	Gradual withdrawal of a patient from dependency.
hemodynamic	Relating to the physical aspects of blood circulation.
protamine	Any of a class of proteins; neutralizes anticoagulant action of heparin.
mediastinal	Relating to the mediastinum (the mass of organs and tissues separating the lungs containing the heart and its large vessels, trachea, esophagus, thymus, lymph nodes, and connective tissue).
Dexon	A synthetic suture material.
apposed	Being placed or fitted together.
autotransfusion	Transfusing back into the body blood that was removed.
exogenous	Originating or produced outside of the organism.

1   PATIENT: Martina Johnson

2   PREOPERATIVE DIAGNOSIS: Coronary artery disease.

3   POSTOPERATIVE DIAGNOSIS: Coronary artery disease.

4   OPERATION: Triple coronary artery bypass grafting
5   (left internal mammary artery bypass to the left
6   anterior descending coronary artery and aortosphenous
7   vein graft to the circumflex obtuse marginal and
8   diagonal branch of the **LAD**).

9   CLINICAL SUMMARY: Mrs. Johnson is a 79-year-old
10   patient of Drs. Burns and Malich who was admitted to
11   the hospital with **epigastric** pain and chest pains. The
12   patient was found to be in **congestive heart failure**.

13   The patient also has a history of **hiatal hernia**.
14   She was transferred to Brookline Hospital where she
15   underwent **cardiac catheterization** and **angiography** which
16   revealed moderately severe **left ventricle dysfunction**,
17   total **occlusion** of the LAD, total occlusion of the
18   right coronary artery, severe **stenosis** of the diagonal
19   and **ostial** stenosis of the left circumflex and
20   midcircumflex obtuse marginal coronary artery. The
21   patient was placed on **intravenous heparin** therapy and
22   referred for urgent coronary **revascularization**.

23   PROCEDURE: With the patient in the **supine** position and
24   under adequate general **endotracheal** anesthesia,
25   the chest and legs were prepped and draped in the usual
26   fashion. The chest was carefully opened with a
27   **median sternotomy**.

28   Veins were removed from the long **saphenous** system of
29   the legs. Veins were prepared at room temperature by
30   flushing and gentle distension with **plasmalyte**
31   containing heparin (1000 units) and **papaverine**
32   (30 mg)/500 cc.

33   Left internal mammary artery was dissected down with
34   **electrocautery** and use of **hemoclips**. It was dilated by
35   injection with papaverine solution containing 30 mg of
36   papaverine in 3 cc of plasmalyte. Free flow was 80 cc
37   to 100 cc/minute.

PATIENT: Martina Johnson
Page 2

38 The **pericardium** was opened and tacked to the **anterior**
39 sternal table and 3 mg/kg of heparin was given. A #20
40 aortic **cannula** and one #51 venous cannula was inserted
41 and bypass begun with a flow rate of 4 to 5
42 liters/minute. Systemic cooling to 25–30°C was carried
43 out. The aorta was crossclamped, and the heart
44 arrested with a cold blood cardioplegic solution
45 (containing 30 mg of potassium per liter of cold blood
46 obtained from the pump at 10°C injected into the
47 aortic root at 200 to 300 cc/minute).

48 When adequate electromechanical arrest was obtained and
49 myocardial temperature was less than 20°C, attention
50 was turned to performance of the **distal anastomoses**.
51 The left anterior descending vein was a 1.5 mm vessel
52 of satisfactory caliber. The diagonal was a 1 mm to
53 1.5 mm thin-walled vessel. The obtuse marginal was a
54 1.5 mm thin-walled vessel. The previously prepared
55 veins were anastomosed to the above-mentioned
56 coronaries using end-to-side connections and running
57 layers of 8-0 Prolene suture.

58 The aorta was unclamped and the heart **defibrillated**.
59 Rewarming to 37°C was carried out.

60 Proximal anastomoses were performed using partial
61 aortic occlusion, linear **arteriotomies**, end-to-side
62 connections and running layers of 7-0 Prolene sutures.
63 After flow was restored to the obstructed coronary
64 system, the patient was **weaned** from bypass.

65 The patient came off bypass without difficulty
66 maintaining satisfactory **hemodynamic** parameters.

67 **Protamine** was given to reverse the heparin. The
68 arterial line and venous cannulae were removed. The
69 usual pacing wires, monitoring lines, and **mediastinal**
70 sumps were inserted; and the pericardium was closed in
71 the midline with **Dexon**. The sternum and soft tissues
72 were **apposed** in the usual fashion, and the patient was
73 taken to the open heart unit.

74 ADDENDUM: Bypass time: 130 minutes.
75 Crossclamp time: 71 minutes (cold blood cardioplegia
76 and profound myocardial hypothermia).

77   Urine on bypass: 250 cc.
78   Blood administered on bypass: 1 unit packed cells.
79   Bypass gradient: 0 cc.

80   A haemonetics **autotransfusion** device was used. As a
81   result, 1 unit of blood was returned to the patient
82   during bypass and 3 units of blood following the
83   discontinuation of bypass. This obviated the need for
84   **exogenous** blood transfusions.

85   _____
86   Patrick Cahill, MD

87   PC/urs

88   d: 7/23/—
89   t: 7/23/—   Word Count 614
90   [cassette]   ORCARMJ.5

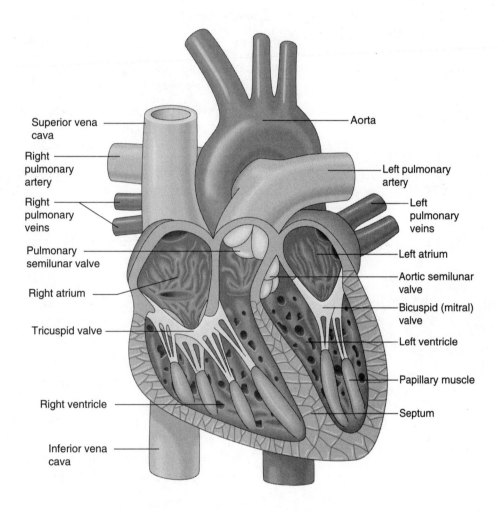

Superior vena cava

Right pulmonary artery

Right pulmonary veins

Pulmonary semilunar valve

Right atrium

Tricuspid valve

Right ventricle

Inferior vena cava

Aorta

Left pulmonary artery

Left pulmonary veins

Left atrium

Aortic semilunar valve

Bicuspid (mitral) valve

Left ventricle

Papillary muscle

Septum

Cross section of the heart

mitral stenosis	Pathologic narrowing of the orifice of the mitral valve.
mitral valve	Valve found between the left atrium and the left ventricle of the heart.
ramus	A branch; one of the dimensions of a forked structure.
RCA	Right coronary artery.
CVA	Cerebrovascular accident (stroke).
ischemic	Relating to or affected by decreased blood flow.
echocardiogram	The ultrasonic record obtained by echocardiography.
cardiac catheterization	A thin tube is introduced into a vein or artery and is guided into the heart for purposes of detecting pressures and patterns of blood flow.
angiography	Radiography of vessels after injection of a radiopaque material.
diuresed	Excreted urine.
Swan-Ganz catheter	A thin, flexible, flow-directed tube using a balloon to carry it through the heart to a pulmonary artery.
intubated	Tube inserted into a canal, hollow organ, or cavity for anesthesia or for control of pulmonary ventilation.
saphenous	Relating to or associated with a saphenous vein; denoting a number of structures in the leg.
heparin	An anticoagulant.
cannulated	An inserted cannula.
cannula	A tube that can be inserted into a cavity, usually by means of a trocar filling its lumen.
vena cavae	Two largest veins in the body.
superior vena cava	Drains blood from the upper portion of the body.
inferior vena cava	Carries blood from the lower part of the body.
cardioplegia	Paralysis of the heart; an elective stopping of cardiac activity temporarily by injection of chemicals, selective hypothermia (the state in which an individual's body temperature is reduced below normal range), or electrical stimuli.
Buckberg-Shiley	A cardioplegic cannula.

antegrade	Moving forward.
retrograde	Moving backward.
saline	A salt solution.
distal	Away from the beginning of a structure.
angiogram	A technique used to define the size and shape of various veins and arteries of organs and tissues.
occluded	Closed, obstructed, or brought together.
thrombus	A clot in the cardiovascular system formed during life from constituents of blood.
debridement	Excision of devitalized tissue and foreign matter from a wound.
mattress sutures	Quilted stitches; utilizing a double stitch that forms a loop about the tissue on both sides of a wound.
atrioventricular	Relating to both the atria and the ventricles of the heart.
catheter	A tubular instrument.
Prolene	A synthetic suture material.
Trendelenburg position	A supine position on the operating table, which is inclined at varying angles so that the pelvis is higher than the head with the knees flexed and legs hanging over the end of the table.
anastomoses	A natural communication between two blood vessels or other structures.
mEq/L	Milliequivalents per liter.
hemodynamic	Relating to the physical aspects of blood circulation.
protamine	Any of a class of proteins; neutralizes anticoagulant action of heparin.
cannulae	Tubes that can be inserted into a cavity, by means of a trocar filling its lumen.
mediastinal	Pertaining to the mediastinum.
approximated	Brought close together.
Dexon	A synthetic suture material.
subcuticular	Pertaining to subepidermic; beneath the outer skin.

1   PATIENT: Paul Hayworth

2   PREOPERATIVE DIAGNOSIS: **Mitral stenosis** and coronary
3   artery disease.

4   POSTOPERATIVE DIAGNOSIS: Mitral stenosis and coronary
5   artery disease.

6   OPERATION: 1) **Mitral valve** replacement (27 mm
7   St. Jude Mitral Valve).

8   2) Double coronary bypass (aortosaphenous
9   vein grafts to the **ramus** intermedius and acute
10   marginal branch of the **RCA**).

11   CLINICAL SUMMARY: This is a 73-year-old male, a
12   patient of Drs. Hyman and Kaufman, who has a history of
13   previous **CVA** two years ago as well as multiple
14   transient **ischemic** episodes over the past couple of
15   years. The patient had an **echocardiogram** which
16   revealed a mass on the mitral valve and evidence of
17   severe mitral stenosis and decreased left ventricular
18   function.

19   The patient underwent **cardiac catheterization** and
20   **angiography** which revealed significant mitral stenosis
21   and coronary artery disease. He had a B-Mode
22   sonography of his carotid arteries which was
23   insignificant for carotid disease.

24   Based on the patient's symptoms and anatomic findings,
25   he was referred for mitral valve replacement and
26   coronary bypass grafting. The patient was scheduled
27   for elective admission to the hospital for valve
28   replacement and coronary bypass grafting but came in
29   emergently because of congestive heart failure. The
30   patient was **diuresed** and optimized for surgery.

31   PROCEDURE: The patient was placed on the operating
32   room table in the supine position. The arterial line
33   and **Swan-Ganz catheter** were placed. The patient was
34   anesthetized, **intubated,** and prepared and draped in
35   the usual fashion for a median sternotomy incision and
36   harvesting of **saphenous** veins from the lower
37   extremities. Simultaneous incisions were made in the
38   lower extremity and sternum. The sternum was split in
39   the midline with a saw. The pericardium was incised and
40   tacked up to the anterior sternal table. The
41   patient was given 3 mg/kg of **heparin** intravenously.

42 The aorta was **cannulated** with a #20 French Bard
43 **cannula**. The right atrium was cannulated with two #34
44 French venous cannulae with the tips directed into the
45 **inferior** and **superior vena cavae,** respectively. A
46 retrograde coronary sinus cannula was inserted via the
47 right atrium into the coronary sinus for delivery of
48 cold blood **cardioplegia** and a **Buckberg-Shiley**
49 cardioplegic cannula was inserted in the aortic root
50 for venting purposes.

51 Cardiopulmonary bypass commenced. The blood
52 temperature was lowered to 30°C and cold blood
53 cardioplegia was delivered both in **antegrade** and
54 **retrograde** fashion. Ice **saline** was poured on the
55 surface of the heart to further decrease myocardial
56 temperature. Attention was given to performance of the
57 **distal** coronary bypass grafts.

58 The right ventricular branch was a 1.5 mm vessel as
59 was the ramus intermedius or first obtuse marginal
60 coronary artery. The **angiogram** showed a totally
61 **occluded** vessel with severely diffuse disease and was
62 not bypassable as was the distal obtuse marginal.

63 A left atriotomy incision was then made. There was no
64 **thrombus** present within the left atrium. The valve was
65 a severely stenotic valve. The anterior leaflet of the
66 mitral valve was excised. The posterior leaflet was
67 left intact. There was some **debridement** of calcium
68 performed. **Mattress sutures** of 2-0 Ethibond
69 pledgeted were placed in a horizontal mattress
70 fashion through the annulus of the mitral valve
71 from the left atrial to the left ventricular side and
72 then brought up through the 27 mm St. Jude mitral
73 valve prosthesis.

74 The valve was seated in position, and the sutures tied
75 in place. A left **atrioventricular catheter** was placed
76 across the valve to keep it incompetent for evacuation
77 of air. The atriotomy incision was closed with 3-0
78 **Prolene** in running fashion as warm blood cardioplegia
79 was given in retrograde fashion. The suture was left
80 untied and snared to the vent catheter.

81 The patient was placed in a steep **Trendelenburg**
82 **position**. The aorta was unclamped and then partially
83 reclamped. The usual maneuvers to remove air were
84 performed. The left atrial ventricular vent was
85 removed, and the suture was tied in place.

86   Echocardiographic confirmation of removal of air was
87   obtained. Once this was confirmed, the partial
88   occluding clamp was placed on the aorta for performance
89   of the proximal aortosaphenous vein **anastomoses**. These
90   were constructed using 6-0 Prolene in running fashion.
91   Air was evacuated from the grafts. Flow was restored,
92   and the partial occluding clamp was removed. Atrial
93   and ventricular pacing wires were placed.

94   Once the patient's temperature reached 36°C and
95   potassium was less than 6 **mEq/L**, he was weaned from
96   cardiopulmonary bypass and maintained satisfactory
97   **hemodynamic** parameters.

98   **Protamine** was given to reverse the heparin. The
99   **cannulae** were removed, and the cannulation sites were
100 oversewn with 4-0 Prolene. A pericardial sump catheter
101 was placed as well as an anterior **mediastinal** chest
102 tube. The mediastinal tissues were approximated in the
103 midline to cover the aorta and the grafts.

104 The sternum was **approximated** with wires. The
105 subcutaneous tissue was closed in two layers with
106 0-Vicryl, and the skin edges approximated with 4-0
107 **Dexon** in **subcuticular** fashion.

108 The patient tolerated the operative procedure and was
109 returned to the open heart unit in critical, but
110 stable condition.

111 ADDENDUM: Bypass time: 168 Minutes.
112 Crossclamp time: 109 Minutes (cold blood cardioplegia
113 and profound myocardial hypothermia).
114 Urine on bypass: 80 cc.
115 Blood administered during bypass: None.
116 Bypass gradient: +120 cc.
117 Valve size and type: 27-mm St. Jude Mitral Valve.

118 _____
119 Vladmir Shapolvsky, MD

120 VS/urs

121 d: 12/13/—
122 t: 12/13/—
123 🔳

Word Count 860
ORCARPH.6

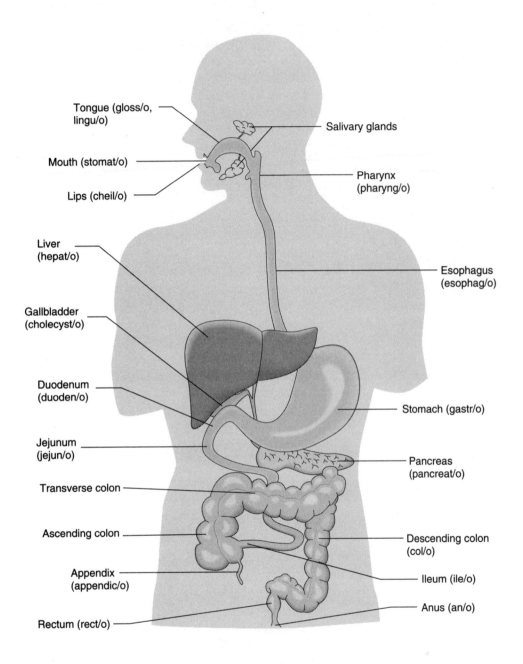

Digestive system

dysphagia	Difficulty swallowing.
esophagogastroduodenoscopy	Inspection of the interior of the lower esophagus, proximal stomach, and duodenum through an endoscope.
percutaneous	Through the outer skin.

PATIENT: Daniella Pestova

SURGEON: Edward Majors, MD

PREOPERATIVE DIAGNOSIS: Chronic nasogastric tube
feeding. **Dysphagia**.

POSTOPERATIVE DIAGNOSIS: Chronic nasogastric tube
feeding. Dysphagia.

OPERATION: **Esophagogastroduodenoscopy**. **Percutaneous**
feeding gastrostomy tube placement.

ANESTHESIA: Versed 2.5 mg IV.

FINDINGS: Esophagus was normal. Fundus and body of
the stomach were normal. Antrum was normal. Pylorus
was normal. The first portion and second portion of the
duodenum were normal.

PROCEDURE: The endoscope was withdrawn into the
stomach, and the catheter was placed percutaneously by
Dr. Edward Majors. A guide wire was inserted through the
catheter which was snared by the endoscope and brought
out through the mouth. The gastrostomy tube was then
threaded over the guide wire with the mushroom head end
lying at the anterior wall of the stomach and the tube
exiting the anterior abdominal wall. The patient was
then re-endoscoped for position, and it was adequate.

IMPRESSION: Normal esophagogastroduodenoscopy and
successful placement of percutaneous feeding
gastrostomy tube.

_____

Edward Majors, MD

EM/urs

d: 7/8/—
t: 7/9/—

Word Count 181
ORGASDP.1

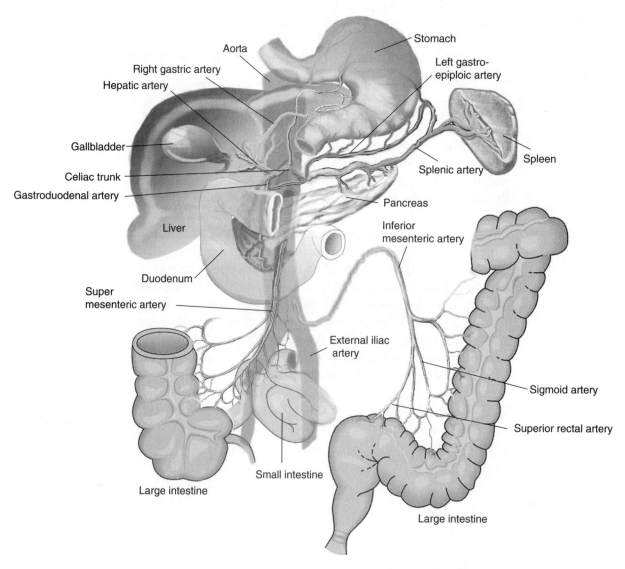

Arterial distribution to organs of the abdominal cavity

stenosis	A stricture or narrowing of any canal or valve.
hepatic duct	Canal that receives bile from the liver. It unites with the cystic duct to form the common bile duct.
biliary	Relating to bile (yellowish brown or green fluid secreted by the liver).
stents	Devices used to maintain a bodily orifice or cavity during skin grafting, or to immobilize a skin graft after placement. Slender thread, rod, or catheter, lying within the lumen of tubular structures, used to provide support during or after their anastomosis, or to assure patency of intact but contracted lumen.
occlusion	The act of closing or the state of being closed.
stasis	Stagnation of normal flow of fluids, as of blood or urine.
fluoroscopic	Relating to or effected by means of fluoroscopy (x-ray).
aspirated	A gas or fluid from a body cavity removed by suction.
duodenum	The first division of the small intestine.
epigastrium	Region over the pit of the stomach.

PUNCTUATION REFERENCES

Line 11	comma—introductory, Rule 7
Line 12	commas—parenthetical, Rule 10
Line 13	semicolon—no conjunction, Rule 1
Line 16	commas—parenthetical, Rule 10
Line 17	semicolon—no conjunction, Rule 1
Lines 18, 19	commas—parenthetical, Rule 10
Line 20	comma—conjunction, Rule 3
Line 22	comma—introductory, Rule 7

1   PATIENT: Norman Keefe

2   PREOPERATIVE DIAGNOSIS: **Stenosis** of the **hepatic duct**.
3   Status post left and right hepatic duct **biliary stents**
4   with stent leak and probable stent **occlusion**.

5   POSTOPERATIVE DIAGNOSIS: Stenosis of the hepatic duct.

6   PATHOLOGY: There was green **stasis** bile in the biliary
7   tree. The stents were occluded.

8   OPERATION: Revision of left and right hepatic duct
9   biliary stents.

10   PROCEDURE: After positioning the patient on the
11   **fluoroscopic** table under sterile precautions, the right
12   hepatic duct, an 8.3 French stent, was **aspirated**. This
13   showed green stasis bile; a sample was sent for
14   culture. Injection of contrast showed the stents to be
15   obstructed with poor flow of contrast into the
16   **duodenum**. The stents were, therefore, entered with a
17   38/100ths straight wire; the left and right hepatic duct
18   stents were removed. A new right hepatic duct, an
19   8.3 French stent, was placed and the wire removed. The
20   biliary tree was then irrigated clear, and the second
21   left hepatic duct was placed through the **epigastrium**. At
22   the completion of the procedure, there was good flow of
23   contrast into the duodenum.

24   The patient tolerated the procedure well and left the
25   x-ray suite in good condition.

26   _____
27   Lester Zimmon, MD

28   LZ/urs

29   d: 6/24/—
30   t: 6/24/—   Word Count 227
31   ▄▄   ORGASNK.2

gastrostomy	Establishment of a new opening into the stomach.
adherent	Attached to, as of two surfaces.
anterior	Front of the body.
ASHD	Arteriosclerotic heart disease.
supine	Lying on the back.
Betadine	Trade name for povidone-iodine, a topical anti-infective.
paramedian	Near the middle line.
subcutaneous	Beneath the skin.
fascia	A fibrous membrane covering, supporting, and separating muscles.
rectus muscles	Two external abdominal muscles, one on each side.
peritoneum	Connective tissue that lines the abdominal cavity and most of the viscera contained therein.
pursestring suture	A continuous stitch placed in a circular manner for either inversion or closure.
Malecot catheter	A two- or four-winged tube with an expanded cup used for gastrotomy feeding.
upper quadrant	Division of the abdomen by a horizontal line and a vertical line intersecting at the umbilicus.

1   PATIENT: Eva Herzigova

2   PREOPERATIVE DIAGNOSIS: **Gastrostomy** tube placement.

3   POSTOPERATIVE DIAGNOSIS: Gastrostomy tube placement.

4   PROCEDURE PERFORMED: Gastrostomy tube insertion.

5   FINDINGS: Stomach **adherent** to **anterior** wall.

6   PROCEDURE: The patient is an 83-year-old female with a
7   history of **ASHD** who presented to the hospital with a
8   gastrostomy tube removed for an unknown amount of time.
9   Attempts at placement in the emergency room failed, and
10   the patient was admitted for reinsertion of the
11   gastrostomy tube.

12   The patient was placed on the operating table in the
13   **supine** position, general anesthesia was induced, and
14   the abdomen was prepped with **Betadine** and draped in the
15   usual sterile manner. A **paramedian** incision was made
16   with a #20 blade and the skin, **subcutaneous** tissue, and
17   **fascia** were incised. The **rectus muscle** was incised and
18   the **peritoneum** was entered by placing clamps on either
19   side. Feeding gastrostomy was performed by placing two
20   rows of **pursestring** 2-0 silk **sutures** in the anterior
21   wall of the stomach. The stomach was incised, and a
22   small **Malecot catheter** introduced. The catheter was
23   brought out through a separate stab wound incision in
24   the **upper quadrant** of the abdomen. The stomach was
25   tacked at the four quadrants to the anterior abdominal
26   wall, and the gastrostomy tube placed with drainage to a
27   Foley bag. The abdomen was closed in layers using
28   interrupted sutures of 2-0 silk. The skin was closed
29   with interrupted mattress sutures of 4-0 silk. Sterile
30   dressings were applied. The patient tolerated the
31   procedure well.

32   Sutures: Silk.   Catheter: #18 feeding tube.
33   Case: Clean.   Specimen: None.

34   Complications: None.   Condition: Good.
35   Drains/Packing: None.

36   _____
37   Helen Kleopoulos, MD

38   HK/urs

39   d: 6/2/—
40   t: 6/2/—   Word Count 282
41   ▣   ORGASEH.3

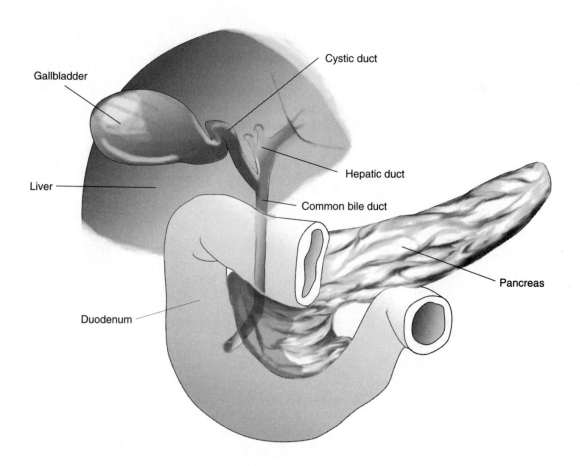

Gallblatter

Cystic duct

Liver

Hepatic duct

Common bile duct

Pancreas

Duodenum

Liver, gallbladder, and pancreas

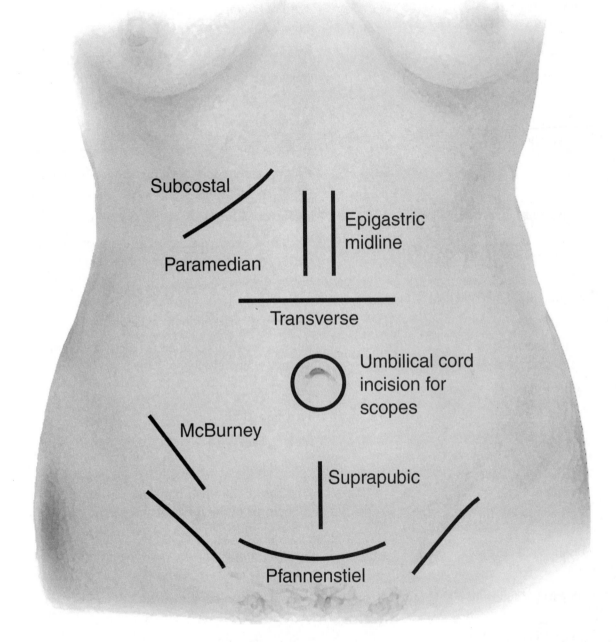

Types of incisions

common bile duct	Duct carrying bile to the duodenum.
cholecystectomy	Surgical removal of the gallbladder.
choledochotomy with T-tube cholangiogram	Surgical incision of the common bile duct with radiographic examination of the common bile duct.
gastrectomy	Surgical removal of a part or all of the stomach.
pruritus	Severe itching.
jaundice	Yellowness of skin, whites of eyes, mucous membranes, and body fluids.
subcostal	Beneath the ribs.
rectus fascia	Fibrous membranes covering supporting rectus abdominal muscles.
transected	Cut across a long axis; a cross section.
posterior fascia	A fibrous membrane covering, supporting, and separating muscles toward the back of the body.
peritoneum	Serous membrane reflected over the viscera and lining of the abdominal cavity.
adhesions	Fibrous bands holding parts together that are normally separated.
cystic duct	Duct of gallbladder.
ligated	Tied/bound off.
retrograde	Moving backward.
dilated	Expanded.
duodenum	First part of the small intestine connecting the pylorus of the stomach and extending to the jejunum.
foramen of Winslow	Opening connecting the peritoneal cavity to its lesser sac.
interrupted figure-of-eight sutures	Utilizing single crisscross stitches fixed by tying ends together.
anterior fascia	Ventral, abdominal fascia.
approximated	Brought close together, closed.

1 PATIENT: Henry Kanter

2 PREOPERATIVE DIAGNOSIS: Impacted stone in **common**
3 **bile duct**.

4 POSTOPERATIVE DIAGNOSIS: Impacted stone in common
5 bile duct.

6 OPERATION: 1. **Cholecystectomy**.

7   2. **Choledochotomy**, **with T-tube cholangiogram**.

8 ANESTHESIA: General. ANESTHESIOLOGIST: Dr. Patrick Rogers.

9   HISTORY: This patient is a 60-year-old male with a
10 past history of partial **gastrectomy** and alcohol abuse.
11 He was admitted this time under the medical service of
12 Dr. Patrick Rogers because of right upper quadrant pain,
13 **pruritus**, and **jaundice**.

14 PROCEDURE: The patient was prepped and draped in the
15 usual manner using sterile technique. A right **subcostal**
16 incision was made. This was carried down to the
17 **rectus fascia** and muscle which were then **transected**.
18 The **posterior fascia** and **peritoneum** were entered.

19 Upon entering the abdomen, there were numerous
20 **adhesions** in the right upper quadrant due to the
21 patient's previous surgery. After careful dissection,
22 the **cystic duct** and artery were identified and were doubly
23 **ligated** and divided. The gallbladder was removed in a
24 **retrograde** fashion. Prior to this, it could be noted
25 that the common bile duct was **dilated,** and there was a
26 large stone in the duct. A choledochotomy was done, the
27 stone was removed, and a #18 T-tube was placed in the
28 common bile duct. The duct was then closed with
29 interrupted sutures of #4-0 Vicryl. A T-tube
30 cholangiogram was done, and two films were taken which
31 showed no residual stone and free flow of contrast into
32 the **duodenum**. The wound was closed after a Jackson-
33 Pratt drain had been placed in the **foramen of Winslow**
34 and brought out through a separate stab wound. The
35 wound was closed using running #0 Vicryl for the
36 peritoneum and posterior fascia and **interrupted figure-**
37 **of-eight** #0 Vicryl for the **anterior fascia**. Skin edges
38 were **approximated** by means of staples.

PATIENT: Henry Kanter
Page 2

39   The patient tolerated the procedure well and left the
40   operating room in good condition.

41

                                              _____

42   Kevin McGrath, MD

43   KM/urs

44   d: 7/27/—
45   t: 7/27/—   Word Count 220
46   ▰   ORGASHK.4

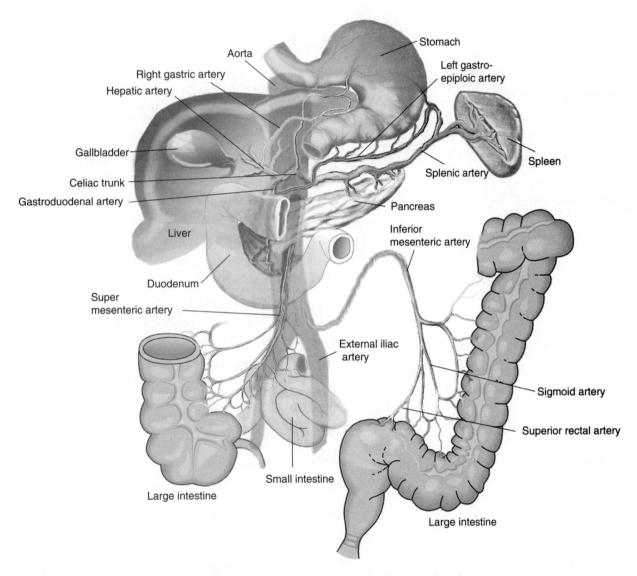

Arterial distribution to organs of the abdominal cavity

abdominal aortic aneurysm	Localized abnormal dilatation of abdominal aorta.
resection	Cutting off/out.
palpable	Able to be felt or touched by hand/fingers.
sonography	Use of ultrasound to produce an image or photograph of an organ or tissue.
hypertension	High blood pressure.
cardiac catheterization	A long, fine, especially designed catheter is passed into the lumen of a blood vessel and into the chambers of the heart.
supine	Flat on the back.
Swan-Ganz catheter	A soft, flexible catheter that contains a balloon near its tip.
intubated	Placement of a tube for air into the larynx or trachea.
peritoneal	Pertaining to the peritoneum (serous membrane over the viscera and lining the abdominal cavity).
mesentery	A peritoneal fold encircling the greater part of the small intestine and connecting the intestines to the posterior abdominal wall.
distal	Farthest from the center.
iliac arteries	Vessels relating to the ilium (one of the bones of each half of the pelvis).
iliac veins	Vessels relating to the ilium.
infrarenal	Below the kidney.
heparin	A solution used to inhibit blood coagulation.
anastomosed	Surgically connected.
hemostasis	Arrest/stop bleeding.
anastomosis	A new surgical connection between segments of an organ.
hemodynamically	Relating to the physical aspects of blood circulation.

1 PATIENT: Salvatore Mino

2 PREOPERATIVE DIAGNOSIS: **Abdominal aortic aneurysm.**

3 POSTOPERATIVE DIAGNOSIS: Abdominal aortic aneurysm.

4 OPERATION: **Resection** of abdominal aortic aneurysm and
5 replacement with a 20-mm Microvel 2 graft.

6 CLINICAL SUMMARY: Mr. Mino is a 70-year-old gentleman
7 who, en route to a physical exam, was found to have a
8 **palpable** abdominal mass. The patient underwent
9 **sonography** which revealed a 5.5-cm abdominal aortic
10 aneurysm. The patient has a history of **hypertension,**
11 contracted pneumonia two years ago, and has smoked a
12 pack of cigarettes a day for 40 years. Based on the
13 patient's physical exam findings, he was determined to
14 be a candidate for abdominal aortic aneurysm resection.

15 He was admitted to the hospital for cardiac evaluation
16 with **cardiac catheterization.** This workup revealed
17 normal coronary arteries with good left ventricular function.

18 PROCEDURE: The patient was placed on the operating
19 table in the **supine** position. Arterial lines and a
20 **Swan-Ganz catheter** were placed. The patient was
21 anesthetized, **intubated,** prepped, and draped in the
22 usual fashion for a midline abdominal incision. The
23 midline abdominal incision was made. The **peritoneal**
24 cavity was entered. Midline retractors were placed. The
25 **mesentery** of the small bowel was separated off of the
26 aorta. **Distal** control of the common **iliac arteries** on
27 both sides was obtained with vessel loops being
28 careful to avoid any injury to the **iliac veins.**
29 Dissection was carried upward. Control of the
30 **infrarenal** abdominal aorta was also obtained. The
31 patient was then given 7500 units of **heparin**
32 intravenously. Both common iliac arteries were clamped
33 followed by clamping of the infrarenal abdominal aorta.

34 The incision was made into the graft. Thrombus was
35 removed. There was one vertebral vessel which was
36 bleeding and that was oversewn with #2-0 silk suture.

37 The proximal aorta was cut in a T-fashion. A 20 mm
38 Microvel graft was **anastomosed** in running fashion using
39 #4-0 Prolene on a C-2 needle. The suture was carried

40   around circumferentially and tied in place. The
41   aortic crossclamp was removed and placed on the graft.

42   **Hemostasis** was satisfactory. The graft was flushed and
43   irrigated with heparinized saline solution. Distally,
44   the incision was carried into the right iliac
45   anteriorly. **Anastomosis** was performed using #4-0 Prolene
46   on a C-2 needle to the distal abdominal aorta with a
47   tongue extending into the right iliac artery.

48   Retrograde bleeding was permitted from both iliacs, and
49   the graft was flushed into the abdominal cavity prior
50   to completion of the suture line. All clamps were
51   removed, and flow was restored independently to each
52   extremity. All suture lines were intact. Hemostasis
53   was satisfactory. The old aortic wall was
54   reapproximated over the graft using #0 Vicryl. The aorta
55   was reperitonealized, and the small bowel was returned
56   to its normal position. The abdomen was closed with
57   interrupted #1 Prolene in Tom Jones' fashion. The skin
58   edges were approximated with staples.

59   The patient was returned to the recovery room in stable
60   condition. The patient remained **hemodynamically** stable
61   throughout the operation.

62
63   _____

                 Dietek Karpinski, MD

64   DK/urs

65   d: 2/3/—
66   t: 2/3/—   Word Count 570
67   ⊟   ORGASSM.5

sacral	Relating to the sacrum.
decubitus	A bedsore; the position of the patient in bed; e.g., dorsal, lateral; sometimes used to refer to a decubitus ulcer.
debridement	The removal of foreign material and dead or damaged tissue.
lateral	Pertaining to the side.
lidocaine	Local anesthetic.
necrotic	Relating to death of a portion of a tissue.
Dakin's solution	A solution for cleansing wounds.
saline	A salt solution.
prosthesis	Fabricated substitute for a diseased or missing part of the body.
suture	A surgical stitch.

1   PATIENT: Sherri Shellooe

2   PREOPERATIVE DIAGNOSIS: Infected **sacral decubitus**.

3   POSTOPERATIVE DIAGNOSIS: Infected sacral decubitus.

4   OPERATION: **Debridement** of infected sacral decubitus.

5   ANESTHESIA: Local, monitored by Dr. Joseph O'Leary.

6   PROCEDURE: The patient was taken to the operating room
7   and placed in the right **lateral** position. The sacral
8   region was draped and prepped in the usual sterile
9   fashion. Utilizing 0.5% **lidocaine** plain local
10   anesthesia, 6 cc, the sacral decubitus was anesthetized
11   at the margins. Using a short scalpel set to
12   220°C, the **necrotic** margin around the sacral decubitus
13   was debrided, and hemostasis was obtained.

14   Wet-to-dry Kerlix with **Dakin's solution** 50% and normal
15   **saline** 50% were packed into the decubitus, and a
16   combined dressing and tape were applied. The patient
17   tolerated the procedure well. There were no complications.

18   Case: Dirty, contaminated. No drains, **prosthesis,**
19   or **suture**.

20   ESTIMATED BLOOD LOSS: 2 cc.

21   FLUID REPLACEMENT: One unit of packed red blood cells
22   and 500 cc of saline.

23   The patient was taken to the postanesthesia recovery
24   room in stable condition.

25   _____

26   Paul Linder, MD

27   PL/urs

28   d: 6/30/—
29   t: 6/30/—   Word Count 179
30   ▪▪▪   ORINTSS.1

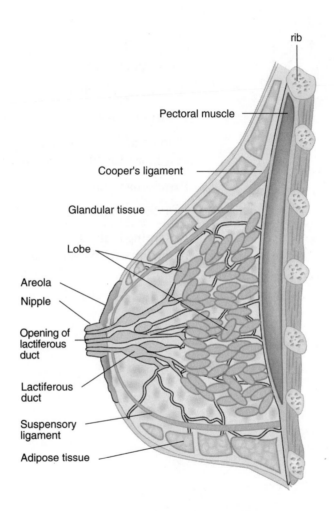

rib

Pectoral muscle

Cooper's ligament

Glandular tissue

Lobe

Areola

Nipple

Opening of
lactiferous
duct

Lactiferous
duct

Suspensory
ligament

Adipose tissue

Sagittal section of female breast

mastectomy	Excision of a breast.
general endotracheal	Production of anesthesia by administering gas inhaled via a tube passed through the trachea.
OR	Operating room.
supine	Flat on the back.
transverse	Crosswise.
superior	Higher than, above.
inferior	Lower than, below.
hemostasis	Arrest/stop bleeding.
pectoralis muscles	Breast muscles.
pectoralis fascia	Fibrous membranes covering, supporting, and separating the pectoralis muscles.
medial	Pertaining to the middle.
lateral	Pertaining to the side.
inferolateral	Pertaining to the side and undersurface of the organ or substructure.

PATIENT: Sheila Tuttle

PREOPERATIVE DIAGNOSIS: Right breast cancer.

POSTOPERATIVE DIAGNOSIS: Right breast cancer.

OPERATION: Right simple **mastectomy**.

ANESTHESIA: **General endotracheal**.

ANESTHESIOLOGIST: Harvey Hicks, MD

FINDINGS: A 2 cm mass right breast at 2 o'clock.

PROCEDURE: Patient was placed on the **OR** table in the **supine** position. After general anesthesia was induced, the patient was prepped and draped in routine sterile fashion. An elliptical **transverse** incision was made around the right breast including the nipple to the level of the anterior ancillary line. Both **superior** and **inferior** skin flaps were raised with sharp dissection. **Hemostasis** was achieved with 3-0 and 2-0 silk ties.

After the flaps were raised, the breast was then taken off the **pectoralis muscles** including the **pectoralis fascia**. After the breast was completely removed from **medial** to **lateral**, hemostasis was again achieved with 2-0 and 3-0 silk sutures. Two Jackson-Pratt drains were placed beneath the skin flaps, and the skin flaps were anchored down to the chest wall using 2-0 chromic sutures.

The Jackson-Pratts were then brought out through separate stab wounds in the **inferolateral** aspect of the wound. The skin edges were then approximated with 3-0 silk interrupted sutures. A dry sterile dressing was placed, and patient was taken to the recovery room in stable condition.

_____

Carl Mishkit, MD

CM/urs

d: 1/23/—
t: 1/23/—
📼

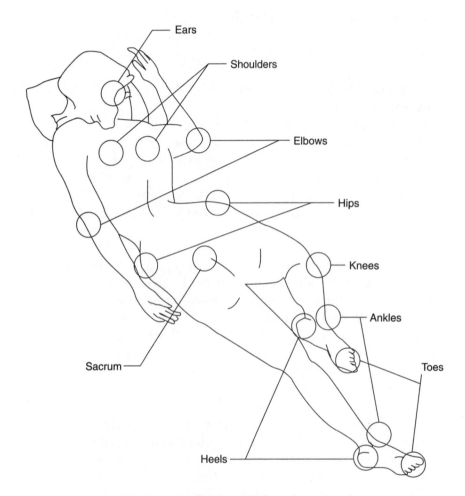

Ears

Shoulders

Elbows

Hips

Knees

Ankles

Toes

Sacrum

Heels

Common sites for decubiti (pressure ulcers)

decubitus ulcer	Ulcer, initially of the skin, due to prolonged pressure over the affected area.
debridement	Removal of dead or damaged tissue.
neuroleptic	General anesthesia produced by the use of a neuroleptic agent such as droperidol, a narcotic analgesic, and nitrous oxide in oxygen.
necrotic	Dead tissue.
prone	Lying facedown.
lidocaine	Local anesthetic.
epinephrine	Adrenaline; used to prolong action of local anesthetics.
periphery	Located away from the center.
hemostasis	Arrest/stop bleeding.
cautery	Used to destroy tissue in potentially infected wounds.

PUNCTUATION REFERENCES

Line 10	commas—series, Rule 1
Line 13	comma—introductory, Rule 7
Line 15	hyphen—compound modifier, Rule 1
Line 16	comma—introductory, Rule 7
Line 20	comma—two-adjective modifier, Rule 2
Line 22	comma—conjunction, Rule 3
Line 25	hyphen—compound modifier, Rule 1
Line 25	comma—conjunction, Rule 3

1 PATIENT: Connie Shute

2 PREOPERATIVE DIAGNOSIS: **Decubitus ulcer** left buttock.

3 POSTOPERATIVE DIAGNOSIS: Decubitus ulcer left buttock.

4 OPERATION: **Debridement** of decubitus ulcer.

5 ANESTHESIA: Local and **neuroleptic**.

6 ESTIMATED BLOOD LOSS: Approximately 10–15 cc.

7 FINDINGS: A deep 4-cm ulcer left buttock with
8 **necrotic** tissue.

9 PROCEDURE: The patient was brought into the operating
10 room, laid **prone** on the table, and prepped and draped
11 over the left buttock region where the left decubitus
12 ulcer was visible. Using 0.5% **lidocaine** with
13 **epinephrine**, the **periphery** of the decubitus ulcer was
14 infiltrated circumferentially with approximately 17 cc
15 total of lidocaine. Using the shell-out knife set to a
16 temperature of 240°C, the decubitus was debrided
17 and excised sharply around its circumference taking
18 several millimeters of skin at the border and debriding
19 down for a distance of about 4 cm total down to good
20 healthy, viable tissue.

21 **Hemostasis** was achieved using the knife as a **cautery**
22 device. Cultures were sent of the decubitus ulcer site,
23 and the specimen was sent of the total decubitus ulcer
24 of the left buttock. The wound was packed using an
25 antibiotic-soaked Kerlix, and the patient was
26 discharged back to her room in good condition.

27 The case was a dirty case. There were no complications.

28 The patient was stable on transfer to her room.

29 _____
30 Frank Pacholka, MD

31 FP/urs

32 d: 1/30/–
33 t: 1/30/–   Word Count 235
34 📼   ORINTCS.3

lesion	A wound or injury; a pathologic change in the tissues; one of the individual points or patches of a multifocal disease.
squamous cell carcinoma	Scaly, malignant cell.
intraoperative	Relating to, or effected within an operation.
excoriated fungating	Grew exuberantly like a fungus or spongy growth scratched or otherwise denuded by the skin by physical means.
occiput	The back of the head.
ulcerated	Of the nature of an ulcer or affected with one.
OR	Operating room.
supine	Lying on the back.
Betadine	Trade name for povidone-iodine, a topical anti-infective.
Xylocaine	Trade name for lidocaine hydrochloride.
calvarium	Skullcap; cerebral cranium.
hemostasis	Arrest/stop bleeding.
electrocautery	An instrument for directing a high-frequency current through a local area of tissue; a metal device heated by an electric current used for burning the skin or other tissues.
ligatures	Threads, wires, fillets, or the like, tied tightly around a blood vessel, the pedicle of a tumor, or other structure to constrict it.
collodion	A protective liquid for cuts or as a vehicle for the local application of medicinal substances.

PUNCTUATION REFERENCES

Line 7	comma—title after a person's name, Rule 7
Line 8	semicolon—no conjunction, Rule 1
Line 10	semicolon—two independent clauses with no coordinating conjunction, Rule 3
Line 10	commas—series, Rule 1
Lines 23, 25	comma—introductory, Rule 7
Line 28	commas—parenthetical, Rule 10
Line 32	comma—introductory, Rule 7
Lines 34, 38, 40	comma—conjunction, Rule 3

1   PATIENT: Michael Wallace

2   PREOPERATIVE DIAGNOSIS: Scalp **lesion**.

3   POSTOPERATIVE DIAGNOSIS: **Squamous cell carcinoma** of
4   the scalp.

5   OPERATION: Excision of squamous cell carcinoma of the scalp.

6   ANESTHESIA: Local with anesthesia standby,
7   Allen Bernstein, MD.

8   Pathology specimen was sent; frozen section revealed
9   squamous cell carcinoma. There were no **intraoperative**
10   complications; all sponge, needle, and instrument
11   counts were correct. Upon examination of the patient's
12   scalp, a 3×3 cm **excoriated fungating** mass was located
13   at the top of **occiput** area. There were no other lesions
14   of the scalp. This lesion was dark brown with **ulcerated**
15   areas in the center.

16   PROCEDURE: The patient was brought to the **OR** and
17   placed on the table in **supine** position. The scalp area
18   was then prepared and painted with **Betadine** solution
19   and draped in the usual sterile fashion. An area of the
20   inner right arm was then prepared with Betadine
21   solution and draped in the usual sterile fashion in
22   case a skin graft was required. Using a 0.5%
23   **Xylocaine** solution, the area of the occiput around the
24   lesion was infiltrated. After the appropriate amount of
25   time, the lesion was then excised sharply around its
26   circumference. This was taken down through the area of
27   the **calvarium**. The lesion was then sent to pathology for
28   official review and, by verbal report of Dr. Ned Oliver,
29   read as squamous cell carcinoma. **Hemostasis** of incision
30   was then obtained using the **electrocautery** device as
31   well as 3-0 silk **ligatures**. After hemostasis was
32   obtained, attention turned to closure.

33   Closure was obtained by the use of deeper layers using
34   interrupted 3-0 chromic sutures, and full-thickness
35   skin was closed using horizontal 3-0 silk mattress
36   sutures. The superficial skin layers were then closed
37   using interrupted 4-0 silk sutures. Gauze and
38   **collodion** dressing were applied to the head, and the

39   procedure was terminated. Patient tolerated the procedure
40   well, and there were no intraoperative complications.

41

42   _____

                           Thomas DelSerra, MD

43   TD/urs

44   d: 1/19/–
45   t: 1/19/–   Word Count 324
46   📼   ORINTMW.4

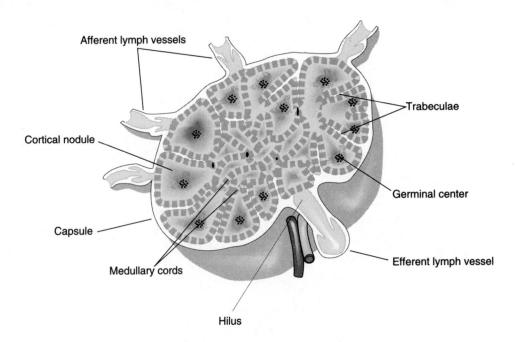

Afferent lymph vessels

Trabeculae

Cortical nodule

Germinal center

Capsule

Efferent lymph vessel

Medullary cords

Hilus

Cross section of a lymph node

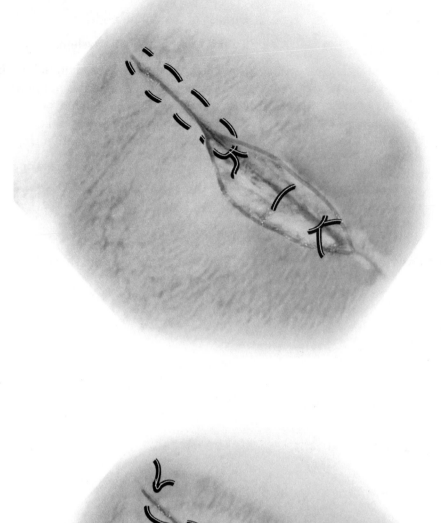

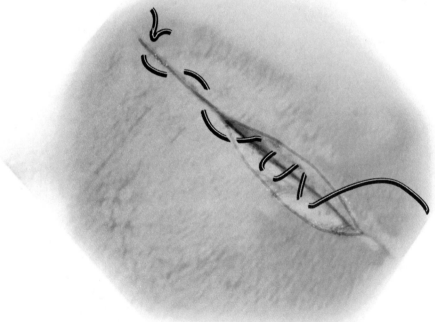

Subcuticular sutures

lymphadenopathy	Disease of the lymph nodes.
lymphoma	Tumor in the lymphatic system.
Scarpa's fascia	Deep layer of superficial abdominal fascia (a fibrous membrane covering, supporting, and separating muscles—it may be deep, enveloping and binding muscles) around edge of the subcutaneous inguinal ring.
areolar	Relating to an areola (a small space or cavity in a tissue).
hemostasis	Arrest/stop bleeding.
excised	Cut out or removed surgically.
subcuticular sutures	Stitches placed through the subcuticular fascia (below the epidermis).

1   PATIENT: Jonathan Lee

2   PREOPERATIVE DIAGNOSIS: Right inguinal
3   **lymphadenopathy**, history of **lymphoma.**

4   POSTOPERATIVE DIAGNOSIS: Right inguinal
5   lymphadenopathy, history of lymphoma, rule out
6   persistent lymphoma.

7   OPERATION: Excision of right inguinal lymph node.

8   ANESTHESIA: Local infiltration of 0.5% lidocaine
9   by Dr. Arthur Clark with Dr. Albert Strong standing by.

10   PATHOLOGY: The patient had a large 3 × 1 cm lymph node
11   in the right inguinal area below **Scarpa's fascia.**

12   PROCEDURE: With the patient in supine position, the
13   right inguinal area was widely prepared with Betadine
14   and draped. After administration of local anesthesia, a
15   transverse incision was made. Incision was carried
16   through Scarpa's fascia with cautery until the lymph
17   node was encountered. The lymph node was then carefully
18   dissected from surrounding vascular and **areolar**
19   attachments. **Hemostasis** was obtained using cautery.
20   Hemostasis was good after the lymph node had been
21   **excised.** The wound was closed in layers using
22   interrupted 3-0 plain catgut to approximate Scarpa's
23   fascia and interrupted 5-0 Vicryl **subcuticular sutures**
24   and 1/8 Steri-strips to approximate the skin. The wound
25   was dressed with Xeroform gauze, dry sterile dressings,
26   and tegaderm.

27   _____
28   Albert Strong, MD

29   AS/urs

30   d: 1/3/—
31   t: 1/3/—   Word Count 203
32   ▄▄   ORLYMJL.1

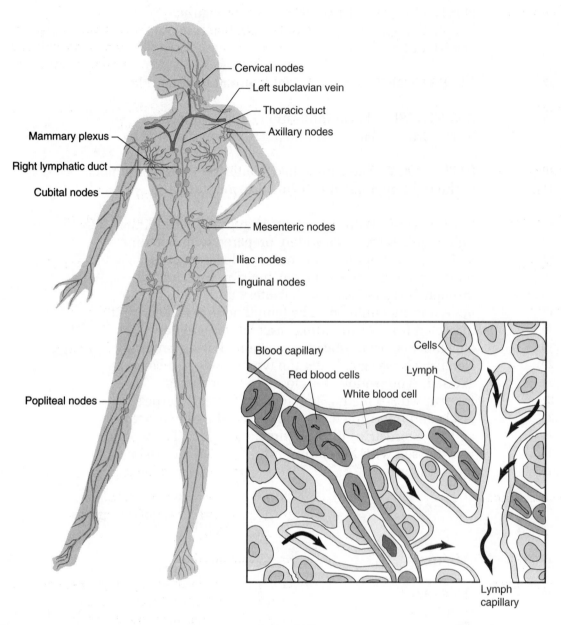

Cervical nodes

Left subclavian vein

Thoracic duct

Axillary nodes

Mammary plexus

Right lymphatic duct

Cubital nodes

Mesenteric nodes

Iliac nodes

Inguinal nodes

Popliteal nodes

Blood capillary

Red blood cells

White blood cell

Cells

Lymph

Lymph capillary

Lymph circulation

edema	An accumulation of an excessive amount of watery fluid in cells, tissues, or serous cavities.
inguinal	Relating to the groin.
lymph node	An encapsulated, rounded body consisting of accumulations of lymphatic tissue. Lymph nodes produce lymphocytes and monocytes and act as filters, keeping bacteria from entering the bloodstream.
biopsy	Excision of a small piece of living tissue for microscopic examination for diagnostic purposes.
supine	Lying on the back.
IV	Intravenous (within a vein).
Ringer's lactate	A sterile solution used intravenously to replace electrolytes.
Betadine	Trade name for povidone-iodine, a topical anti-infective.
palpated	Examined by feeling and pressing with the palms of the hands and the fingers.
infiltrated	Penetration of a substance into a cell or tissue; solution injected into tissues.
lidocaine	Local anesthetic.
transverse	Crosswise.
lateral	Pertaining to the side.
femoral	Relating to the femur or thigh.
Scarpa's fascia	The deeper, membranous part of the subcutaneous tissue of the lower abdominal wall.
hemostasis	Arrest/stop bleeding.
electrocautery	An instrument for directing a high-frequency current through a local area of tissue; a metal cauterizing instrument heated by an electric current.
pedicle	A stem to which a new growth attaches.

1   PATIENT: Natalie Tucker

2   PREOPERATIVE DIAGNOSIS: Tuberculosis and right lower
3   leg **edema**.

4   POSTOPERATIVE DIAGNOSIS: Tuberculosis and right lower
5   leg edema.

6   OPERATION: Right **inguinal lymph node biopsy**.

7   ANESTHESIA: Local.

8   PROCEDURE: The patient was brought into the operating
9   room, placed in the **supine** position, and an **IV** was
10   started, 20 gauge in the right arm, with **Ringer's**
11   **lactate** running at approximately 50 cc per hour.

12   The patient was prepped first by shaving the right
13   groin area. The area was then prepped with **Betadine** and
14   draped in a sterile manner. Right inguinal area was then
15   **palpated** and **infiltrated** with local anesthesia,
16   **lidocaine** 1% without epinephrine. A **transverse** incision,
17   approximately 4 cm, was made below the right inguinal
18   area **lateral** to the **femoral** artery and the vein.
19   The incision was carried through **Scarpa's fascia**.
20   **Hemostasis** was achieved using **electrocautery** and using
21   4-0 Vicryl.

22   The lymph node was identified and sharply dissected
23   free from its **pedicle** using 4-0 Vicryl ties, and
24   hemostasis was achieved again using 4-0 Vicryl ties and
25   electrocautery. After hemostasis was achieved and the
26   lymph node was taken out, the space was closed by using 4-0
27   Vicryl closing Scarpa's fascia in a continuous running
28   stitch. The skin was closed using 4-0 nylon interrupted
29   simple sutures.

30   The wound was then cleansed and dried. A Xeroform gauze
31   was placed over the wound, and dry sterile dressing was
32   applied. The patient tolerated the procedure well and
33   was awake and alert. She complained of minor discomfort in
34   the right groin area. The patient was taken to the

PATIENT: Natalie Tucker
Page 2

35 holding area in the operating room and then transferred
36 to the floor.

37 _____
38   Umberto Sohn, MD

39 US/urs

40 d: 12/10/—
41 t: 12/10/—   Word Count 280
42 ▛▟   ORLYMNT.2

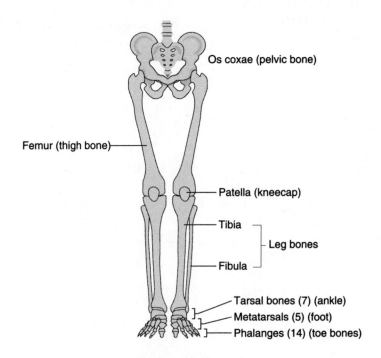

Os coxae (pelvic bone)

Femur (thigh bone)

Patella (kneecap)

Tibia
Fibula
Leg bones

Tarsal bones (7) (ankle)
Metatarsals (5) (foot)
Phalanges (14) (toe bones)

Bones of the lower extremity

scalpel	A knife used in surgical dissection.
fascial	Pertaining to the fascia (a fibrous membrane covering, supporting, and separating muscles).
hemostasis	Arrest/stop bleeding.
lipomatous	Affected with lipoma (fatty tumor).
excised	Cut out surgically.
subcutaneous	Beneath the skin.
subcuticular	Beneath the epidermis.
interrupted sutures	Sutures formed by single stitches inserted separately and fixed by tying ends together.
crystalloid	Resembling a crystal.

1	PATIENT: Judith Bryden
2	PREOPERATIVE DIAGNOSIS: Mass in the left thigh.
3	POSTOPERATIVE DIAGNOSIS: Mass in the left thigh.
4	OPERATION: Removal of mass from left thigh.
5	ANESTHESIA: General.

6 PROCEDURE: The left thigh and leg were prepped and
7 draped in the usual manner. Using a #15 blade
8 **scalpel,** an approximate 5-cm incision was made in a
9 vertical manner. Dissection was carried down to the
10 mass over the **fascial** layer using Metzenbaums.

11 **Hemostasis** was obtained using 3-0 silk sutures. Then
12 the mass was removed. The mass was approximately
13 2 × 2 cm and was a **lipomatous-**type mass. It was **excised**
14 completely off the fascial layer. The 2-cm fascial
15 defect was closed using 3-0 silk × 3. The **subcutaneous**
16 layer was closed with 3-0 silk interrupted layers.
17 The skin was closed using 3-0 silk sutures; **subcuticular**
18 **interrupted sutures** were placed ×5. Then the skin
19 was closed using 4-0 silk interrupted sutures.
20 Approximately eight sutures were used.

21 A dressing was applied. The patient tolerated the
22 procedure well without complications. There was
23 minimal bleeding. Fluid was 100 cc of **crystalloid**.

24 The patient was transferred to the recovery room in
25 stable condition.

26 The patient was discharged to home on a regular diet
27 with regular activities and is to be followed up at my
28 office next Thursday, March 17, 20–.

29 _____
30 Stanley Nealon, MD

31 SN/urs

32 d: 3/10/–
33 t: 3/10/–   Word Count 231
34   ORMUSJB.1

osteomyelitis	Inflammation of bone, especially the marrow.
metatarsal	Metatarsal arch of the foot.
lidocaine	Local anesthetic.
lateral	Pertaining to the side.
flexor tendon	Connective tissue that attaches the flexor muscle (bends a part in a generally proximal direction) to bones and other parts; opposed to extensor.
extensor tendon	Connective tissue that attaches the extensor muscle (extends a part) to bones and other parts.
digital arteries and veins	Arteries and veins in the toe.
ligated	Tied/bound off.
rongeur	An instrument for removing small amounts of tissue, particularly bone.
hemostasis	Arrest/stop bleeding.
sutures	Surgical stitches.
iodoform gauze	Gauze containing a mild antibacterial agent.

1 PATIENT: Michele Valdez

2 PREOPERATIVE DIAGNOSIS: **Osteomyelitis** right fifth
3 **metatarsal**.

4 POSTOPERATIVE DIAGNOSIS: Osteomyelitis right
5 fifth metatarsal.

6 OPERATION: Amputation of right fifth toe and metatarsal.

7 ANESTHESIA: Regional block using 0.5% **lidocaine** by
8 Fred Bernstein, MD.

9 ESTIMATED BLOOD LOSS: Approximately 50–100 cc.

10 SPECIMENS: Right fifth toe and metatarsal.

11 COMPLICATIONS: None.

12 PROCEDURE: The patient was prepped and draped over the
13 right foot area. The regional block was placed into
14 the foot using 0.5% lidocaine by Dr. Bernstein. The
15 foot was prepped and draped exposing the right foot.

16 Using #10 blade, an incision was made around the fifth
17 toe and down the **lateral** aspect of the foot to the
18 level of the proximal metatarsal joint. The incision
19 was taken down sharply dividing the **flexor** and **extensor**
20 **tendons** of the toe. The **digital artery** and **veins** were
21 **ligated** using #3-0 silk, and the soft tissue was cut
22 back to the level of the proximal metatarsal bone of
23 the fifth digit. The bone was cut at the proximal tip
24 of the metatarsal using a bone cutter and **rongeur** to
25 smooth out the edges and more **hemostasis** was achieved
26 using #3-0 ties. The lateral aspect of the incision on the
27 lateral aspect of the foot was closed using two interrupted
28 **sutures** of #3-0 wire. The rest of the wound was left
29 open and packed with **iodoform gauze** and dressed
30 with Kerlix wrap. The patient tolerated the procedure
31 well and was discharged in good condition without
32 any complications.

33   _____
34   Shirley Pacholka, MD

35 SP/urs

36 d: 6/15/—
37 t: 6/15/—   **Word Count 259**
38 📼   ORMUSMV.2

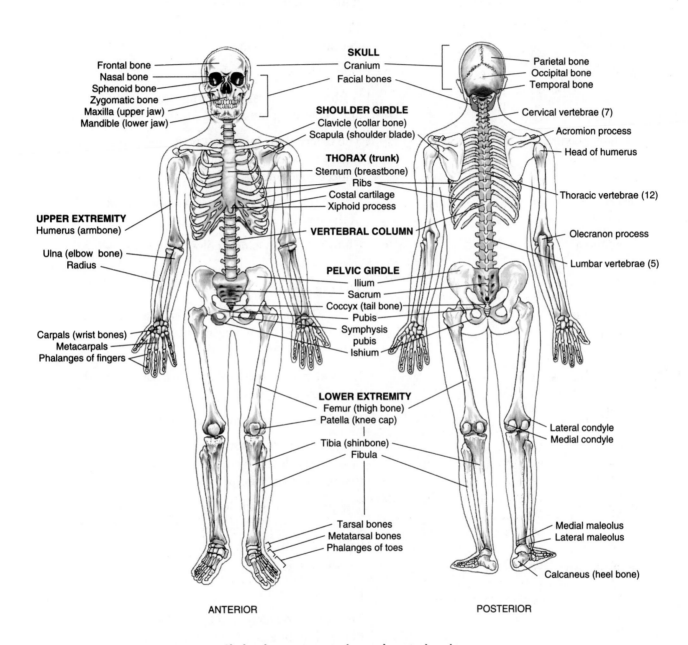

SKULL
Cranium
Facial bones

Frontal bone
Nasal bone
Sphenoid bone
Zygomatic bone
Maxilla (upper jaw)
Mandible (lower jaw)

Parietal bone
Occipital bone
Temporal bone

Cervical vertebrae (7)
Acromion process
Head of humerus

SHOULDER GIRDLE
Clavicle (collar bone)
Scapula (shoulder blade)

THORAX (trunk)
Sternum (breastbone)
Ribs
Costal cartilage
Xiphoid process

Thoracic vertebrae (12)

VERTEBRAL COLUMN

UPPER EXTREMITY
Humerus (armbone)

Olecranon process

Lumbar vertebrae (5)

Ulna (elbow bone)
Radius

PELVIC GIRDLE
Ilium
Sacrum
Coccyx (tail bone)
Pubis
Symphysis
pubis
Ishium

Carpals (wrist bones)
Metacarpals
Phalanges of fingers

LOWER EXTREMITY
Femur (thigh bone)
Patella (knee cap)

Lateral condyle
Medial condyle

Tibia (shinbone)
Fibula

Tarsal bones
Metatarsal bones
Phalanges of toes

Medial maleolus
Lateral maleolus

Calcaneus (heel bone)

ANTERIOR

POSTERIOR

Skeletal system: anterior and posterior views

open reduction	In orthopedics, realigning the fractured segments after incising the skin and tissues in order to expose the fractured bone.
prosthesis	Replacement of a missing part by an artificial substitute.
lateral	Pertaining to the side.
posterior	Dorsal; back of the body.
fascia	A fibrous membrane covering, supporting, and separating muscles.
gluteus maximus	The external prominences posterior to the hips. Formed by the gluteal muscles and underlying structures.
greater trochanter	One of the major bony processes below the neck of the femur.
hematoma	Clotted or partly clotted blood caused by a break in a blood vessel.
femur	The thigh bone.
acetabulum	A cup-shaped depression on the external surface of the hip bone, in which the head of the femur fits.
debrided	Excised foreign material and dead or damaged tissue from a wound.
medullary	Relating to the medulla or marrow.
curet	Instrument in the form of a loop, ring, or scoop with sharpened edges attached to a rod-shaped handle.
impaction	The process or condition of being wedged or pressed closely together so as to be immovable; overload of an organ.
hemostasis	Arrest/stop bleeding.
supine	Lying on the back.
abduction	The lateral movement of the limbs away from the median plane of the body.

1 PATIENT: John Giblin

2 PREOPERATIVE DIAGNOSIS: Fracture of left hip.

3 POSTOPERATIVE DIAGNOSIS: Fracture of left hip.

4 OPERATION: **Open reduction** and Thompson **prosthesis** of
5 left hip (1-7/8%).

6 ANESTHESIA: Spinal.

7 PROCEDURE: Under satisfactory spinal anesthesia, the
8 patient was placed on the operating table in the right
9 **lateral** position with the left hip pointing up. The
10 extremity was prepped and draped in the usual fashion.
11 The hip joint was approached through a **posterior**
12 Austin-Moore approach. The incision was deepened to
13 reach the **fascia** which was cut in the line of incision
14 exposing the **gluteus maximus** muscle which was split in
15 the line of incision. The extremity was brought into
16 internal rotation, and the attachment of the short
17 lateral rotator muscles to the pit of the **greater**
18 **trochanter** was sharply incised. The posterior capsule
19 was incised in a T-shaped manner, and capsular flaps
20 were developed. The fracture site was identified, and
21 the **hematoma** evacuated. The head of the **femur** was
22 extracted from the **acetabulum** with a corkscrew and the
23 hematoma was **debrided** as necessary.

24 The **medullary** canal of the femur was brought into
25 view which was first identified with a **curet** and
26 further developed with a rasp. A 1-3/4 inch Thompson's
27 prosthesis was selected for replacement, and the stem
28 part of the prosthesis was inserted into the previously
29 prepared medullary canal. After proper **impaction,** the
30 head of the prosthesis was reduced into the acetabulum,
31 and the joint was tested for range of motion and stability,
32 both of which were found to be satisfactory. The wound
33 was then thoroughly irrigated.

34 **Hemostasis** was achieved and closed in layers in routine
35 fashion. Sterile dressings were placed over the wound,
36 and the patient was returned to the **supine** position. An
37 **abduction** brace was applied to keep the operated extremity
38 in 30 degrees of abduction. A single x-ray taken in the
39 3 anteroposterior position revealed excellent placement

40 of the Thompson's prosthesis. The patient was returned
41 to the recovery room in satisfactory condition.

42

43 _____

      David S. Bhupathi, MD

44 DSB/urs

45 d: 7/26/—
46 t: 7/26/—   Word Count 348
47   ORMUSJG.3

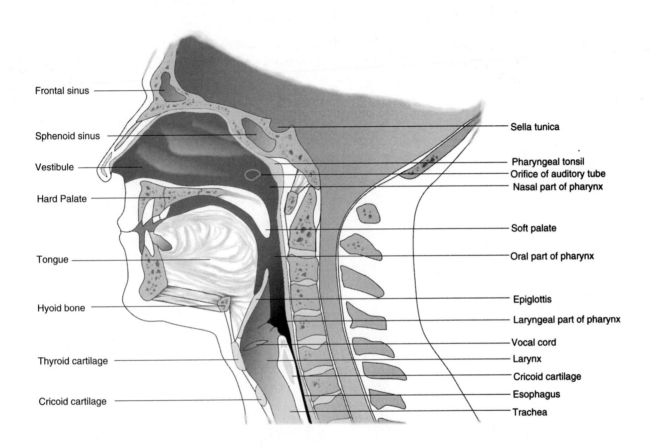

Frontal sinus

Sphenoid sinus

Vestibule

Hard Palate

Tongue

Hyoid bone

Thyroid cartilage

Cricoid cartilage

Sella tunica

Pharyngeal tonsil
Orifice of auditory tube
Nasal part of pharynx

Soft palate

Oral part of pharynx

Epiglottis

Laryngeal part of pharynx

Vocal cord

Larynx

Cricoid cartilage

Esophagus

Trachea

Sagittal section of the face and neck

ORRESMJ.1	Michael Jules	Terminology Preview
microlaryngoscopy		Examination of the interior of the larynx with a small laryngoscope.
in situ		In position, localized; in the normal place without disturbing or invading the surrounding tissue.
laryngoscopy		Examination of the interior of the larynx.
aryepiglottic		Pertaining to the arytenoid cartilage and the epiglottis.
erythematous		Relating to or marked by erythema (inflammatory redness of the skin).

1   PATIENT: Michael Jules

2   PREOPERATIVE DIAGNOSIS: Right vocal cord lesion.

3   POSTOPERATIVE DIAGNOSIS: Right vocal cord lesion.

4   OPERATION: Direct suspension **microlaryngoscopy**. Right
5   vocal cord stripping.

6   FINDINGS: This is a gentleman who has a history of a
7   right vocal cord carcinoma **in situ** which was stripped
8   approximately two years ago. He has a chronically
9   inflamed right vocal cord which was not responsive to
10   medical therapy over the last several months.

11   PROCEDURE: The patient was prepped and draped in the
12   usual manner under adequate general anesthesia. The
13   **laryngoscopy** was performed. Examination of the base of
14   the tongue and **aryepiglottic** fold all appeared to be
15   within normal limits. There was a slightly **erythematous**
16   region on the surface on the middle and posterior
17   surface of the right vocal cord. Complete right vocal cord
18   stripping was performed. The patient tolerated the
19   procedure well and left the operating room awake and
20   in good condition.

21

22   Ada Valez, MD

23   AV/urs

24   d: 6/10/–
25   t: 6/11/–   Word Count 179
26   ■▬   ORRESMJ.1

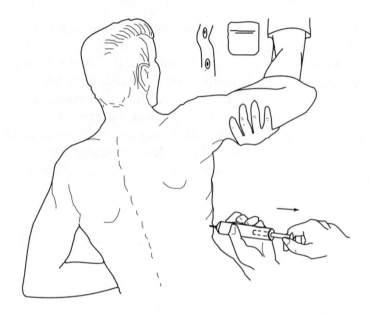

Thoracentesis: removing fluid from the pleural cavity

pleural effusion	Fluid in thoracic cavity between the visceral and parietal pleura.
thoracentesis	Surgical puncture of chest wall for removal of fluid.
posterior	Dorsal, toward the back.
lidocaine	Local anesthetic.
epinephrine	Extract used to relax bronchioles.
midscapular	Center of scapula.
infiltrated	Passed through.
puncture site	Location/place of hole or wound.
post-thoracentesis	Following a thoracentesis procedure.
pneumothorax	Collapse of the lung.
ASU	Ambulatory surgical unit.

1   PATIENT: Patrick Attardi

2   PREOPERATIVE DIAGNOSIS: Left **pleural effusion**.

3   POSTOPERATIVE DIAGNOSIS: Left pleural effusion.

4   OPERATION: Left **thoracentesis**.

5   PROCEDURE: The patient was brought into the operating
6   room, positioned sitting on the table, and leaning
7   forward onto a Mayo stand with pillows to make him
8   comfortable. The left back was prepped and draped over
9   a marker that had been placed on the left **posterior**
10 chest prior to x-ray to mark the level of the pleural
11 effusion and using 1% **lidocaine,** without **epinephrine**, an
12 area of the skin was anesthetized.

13 The patient had approximately 35 cc over the eighth
14 **midscapular** line in the left posterior chest. Using a
15 #22 needle, the pleural space was **infiltrated,** and
16 approximately 100 to 120 cc of straw-colored pleural
17 fluid was extracted. The needle was removed with a
18 small dressing placed over the left back **puncture**
19 **site**. A pleural fluid sample was sent for appropriate
20 studies, and the patient was sent down for a **post-**
21 **thoracentesis** chest x-ray which revealed no **pneumothorax**
22 and decreased pleural effusion. The patient tolerated
23 the procedure well and was discharged back to the
24 **ASU** recovery room. He was sent home later that morning
25 in good condition.

26 _____
27 Agnes Walsh, MD

28 AW/urs

29 d: 1/24/—
30 t: 1/24/—

Word Count 216
31 ⬛

ORRESPA.2

Foley catheter	Urinary tract catheter.
CVP line	Central venous pressure line.
scapula	Shoulder blade.
T2	Second thoracic vertebra.
lateral	Pertaining to the side.
deltoid	Triangular-shaped (deltoid muscle covers the shoulder prominence).
intubated	Tube inserted into the larynx.
hemothorax	Bloody fluid in the pleural cavity.
pneumothorax	A collection of air or gas in the pleural cavity.
IJ line	Internal jugular (cardiovascular) line.
pelvis	Massive cup-shaped ring of bone at the lower end of the trunk.
dorsum	Back or posterior part.
metacarpals	Bones of the hands.
extubated	Removal of tube (see intubated above).
intrathoracic	Within the chest/thorax.

1   PATIENT: Donald Briggs

2   PREOPERATIVE DIAGNOSIS: Gunshot wound in the back.

3   POSTOPERATIVE DIAGNOSIS: Gunshot wound in the back.

4   ESTIMATED BLOOD LOSS: Minimal.

5   FLUIDS PER LITER: **Foley catheter** was 200 cc.

6   OPERATION: 1. Repair of laceration right hand.

7   2. Insertion of left **CVP line.**

8   3. Insertion of Foley catheter.

9   HISTORY AND PROCEDURE: This is a 25-year-old male
10   found at the scene of a burglary and shot in the back.
11   The entrance wound was between the **scapula** at the level
12   of approximately **T2** and an exit wound to the
13   **lateral** aspect of the left **deltoid** in the upper arm.

14   The patient was brought to the operating room and
15   had stable vital signs throughout. In the operating
16   room, he was **intubated** with a crash intubation
17   technique. He then had an x-ray which showed no **hemo-**
18   or **pneumothorax**. He had a left **IJ line** placed with a
19   CVP of 7–8 range. He had a repeat chest x-ray which
20   confirmed the position and which showed no change in the
21   hemothorax. Lateral cervical spine was done to rule
22   out any bullets. The **pelvis** was done which was
23   negative x-ray. The right hand was actively bleeding
24   from a wound in the **dorsum** between the first
25   and second **metacarpals**, and this was irrigated
26   and closed with a running nylon stitch. The patient
27   then had a Foley catheter inserted. A clear urine
28   sample was sent for micro. The patient was **extubated**
29   in the operating room and appeared to have no
30   **intrathoracic** damage from the bullet. The right
31   hand was elevated and appeared stable. The patient was

32   brought to the recovery room in stable condition. At
33   that point the patient agreed with the care he
34   would follow.

35
36   _____

                                              Robert O'Hea, MD

37   RO/urs

38   d: 3/24/—
39   t: 3/24/—   **Word Count 304**
40   ▆▆   **ORRESDB.3**

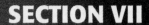

Discharge Summary Reports

OVERVIEW

In this section the student will be transcribing discharge summary reports specific to the cardio-vascular, endocrine, female reproductive, gastrointestinal, genitourinary, musculoskeletal, nervous, respiratory, and special sense body systems.

Terminology previews are provided for each report. Punctuation references illustrating uses of the hyphen, comma, apostrophe, and semicolon are provided in four reports.

DISCHARGE SUMMARY REPORTS

Discharge summary reports are prepared on every patient discharged from a hospital. The report records significant aspects of the patient's medical history, laboratory tests performed, course of treatment while in the hospital, discharge diagnosis, and condition on discharge. Other sections of the discharge summary will be included according to the physician's instructions.

Use of a Macro

It is recommended that the student prepare a macro on a word processor to contain the heading, DISCHARGE SUMMARY, and the side headings for PATIENT:, CHART #:, ADMITTED:, and DISCHARGED (as shown in the transcribed reports). The macro can be named and retrieved with "Alt d." (Consult your instructional manual for macro preparation, as needed.)

Multiple Page Headings

When the report exceeds one page, key the patient's name, chart number, and page number beginning on the first line of each succeeding page. For example,

Loretta Edwards

#123 456

Page 2

Saving and Coding Transcripts

The student should name and save each transcribed report with the code provided at the end of each report.

INSTRUCTIONAL OBJECTIVES

In this chapter, the student will:

1. Transcribe discharge summary reports of varying lengths.
2. Learn terminology relative to the cardiovascular, endocrine, female reproductive, gastrointestinal, genitourinary, musculoskeletal, nervous, respiratory, and special sense body systems.
3. Reinforce understanding of the use of the comma (introductory words and phrases, series, apposition, parenthetical, two-adjective modifiers, date and year, and conjunction), semicolon (when second independent clause contains commas), hyphen (compound modifier, certain adjective forms), and apostrophe (singular possessive).

REMINDERS: Preview highlighted medical terms and punctuation references in the report.
Listen to the tape to become familiar with it.
Transcribe the report inserting punctuation "cues."
Print out a hard copy.
Check carefully your transcribed report word by word to the text transcript.

THE TRANSCRIPT IN THE TEXT IS CHECKED <u>ONLY AFTER</u> YOU HAVE COMPLETED YOUR TRANSCRIPTION.

Record the number of lines transcribed and the number of minutes needed to complete the report.
Make corrections; submit the corrected transcript to your instructor.

DISCHARGE SUMMARY REPORTS INDEX

	Patient Name	Code Name	Word Count
CAR	HERB CANNONS	DSCARHC.1*	259
	MICHAEL SMYTHE	DSCARMS.2	422
END	LOUISE RASKIN	DSENDLR.2	249
FEM	YOLANDA GUOBADIA	DSFEMYG.1	160
	EUGENIA ROMAN	DSFEMER.2	233
	DOROTHY SUTTON	DSFEMDS.3	241
GAS	JULIE WRIGHT	DSGASJW.1	289
	MARGARET LYNCH	DSGASML.2	305
	DMITRIY KAMENSHICH	DSGASDK.3	370
	SYLVIA HIRSCH	DSGASSH.4	358
	MARILYN YOUNG	DSGASMY.5	356
	GEORGE DILORENZO	DSGASGD.6	441
GEN	HERBERT JONES	DSGENHJ.1*	149
	ETTA FARTHINGS	DSGENEF.2	312
	CLIFF MORTON	DSGENCM.3	416
	YOSHIE TAKAHASHI	DSGENYT.4	456
MUS	DAVID LOPEZ	DSMUSDL.2*	243
	FRANK AARON	DSMUSFA.3	510
NER	VALERIE SULLIVAN	DSNERVS.1	148
	IRENA SVETSKY	DSNERIS.2	317
RES	STANLEY STAPLES	DSRESSS.1*	442
SEN	SUSAN ROSS	DSSENSR.1	424

*Punctuation References

myocardial infarction		Necrosis (the death of areas of tissue or bone surrounded by healthy parts) of the cells of an area of the heart muscle (myocardium) caused by oxygen deprivation, in turn caused by obstruction of the blood supply (commonly called a "heart attack").
thrombolytic		Dissolving or splitting up a thrombus (a blood clot that obstructs a blood vessel or a cavity of the heart).
tPA		Tissue-type plasminogen activator (protocol for use in myocardial infarction patients).
CCU		Cardiac care unit.
atrial fibrillation		A cardiac arrhythmia (irregularity or loss of rhythm of the heartbeat) marked by rapid, randomized contractions of the atrial myocardium, causing a totally irregular, often rapid, ventricular rate.
antiarrhythmic		Preventing or alleviating cardiac arrhythmias.
DC		Direct current.
cardioversion		The restoration of normal rhythm of the heart by electrical shock.
ambulating		Walking.
catheterization		Passage of a catheter into a body channel or cavity.
CPK		Creatine phosphokinase (kinase—an enzyme that catalyzes the transfer of phosphate from ATP [adenosine triphosphate] to an acceptor).
MB		Measurement of creatine phosphokinase isoenzyme MB bands of cardiac muscle.

PUNCTUATION REFERENCES

Line 4	hyphens—compound modifier, Rule 1
Line 15	comma—introductory phrase, Rule 7
Line 22	hyphen—compound modifier, Rule 1
Lines 28, 29	commas—series, Rule 1
Lines 31, 32	commas—series, Rule 1
Line 33	apostrophe—singular possessive, Rule 1

| 1 | PATIENT: Herb Cannons | ADMITTED: 10/18/– |
| 2 | CHART #: | DISCHARGED: 10/24/– |

3 HISTORY:
4 The patient is a 71-year-old male admitted for an acute
5 **myocardial infarction** of the anteroseptal wall. He was
6 given **thrombolytic** therapy consisting of **tPA** and put on
7 **CCU** protocol.

8 HOSPITAL COURSE:
9 The patient was noted to be in **atrial fibrillation** with
10 a moderate to rapid ventricular response. He was put
11 on class I **antiarrhythmic** therapy and anticoagulation
12 therapy to convert to normal sinus rhythm.

13 The patient was attempted at **DC cardioversion** ×3
14 to no avail. He remained in atrial fibrillation.

15 While on anticoagulation therapy, he had multiple
16 episodes of retrosternal chest pains on mild to
17 moderate exertion while **ambulating** in the room.

18 The patient was advised to have urgent transfer to
19 Brookfield University Hospital for cardiac
20 **catheterization** to rule out significant coronary
21 artery disease.

22 The patient was noted to have non-insulin dependent
23 diabetes mellitus, and he was put on Accu-Checks and
24 DiaBeta. He had prompt recovery with these dosages
25 with **CPKs** well over 1000 with positive **MB** fractions.
26 EKG revealed anteroseptal wall myocardial infarction
27 with nonspecific ST-T wave changes and atrial
28 fibrillation. The patient was put on beta blockade,
29 nitrate therapy with nitroglycerin, and heparin drip.

30 He is being transferred to Brookfield University
31 Hospital for cardiac catheterization. The risks,
32 benefits, and alternatives were explained to the
33 patient's family members, and they have consented to
34 his transfer to Brookfield University Hospital.

35 _____
36 David Bethaney, MD

37 DB/urs

38 d: 10/24/–
39 t: 10/25/– Word Count 259
40 DSCARHC.1

CABG	Coronary artery bypass graft.
claudication	Limping or lameness.
ambulation	Ability to walk.
angina	Spasmodic, choking, or suffocative pain; now used almost exclusively to denote angina pectoris (severe pain around the heart caused by a relative deficiency of oxygen supply to the heart muscle).
palpitations	A heartbeat that is unusually rapid.
ETOH (ethanol—ethyl alcohol consumption/dependency)	Alcoholic (chemical dependency).
carotid	Relating to the carotid artery, the principal artery of the neck.
radial	Pertaining to the radius of the arm or to the radial (lateral) aspect of the arm as opposed to the ulnar (medial) aspect.
brachial	Pertaining to the arm.
femoral	Pertaining to the femur or to the thigh.
popliteal	Pertaining to the area behind the knee.
dorsalis pedis	Pertaining to the back of the foot.
tibial	Pertaining to the inner and larger bone of the leg between the knee and the ankle.
guaiac positive	Abnormal condition. (An alcoholic solution of guaiac is used for testing occult blood in feces.)
melanotic	Unusual deposit of dark pigment in a body part.
SFA	Superficial femoral artery.
posterior tibialis	Concerning the back of the tibia.
BE	Barium enema.

1	PATIENT: Michael Smythe	ADMITTED: 10/7/–
2	CHART #:	DISCHARGED: 10/11/–

3 CHIEF COMPLAINT:
4 Right and left leg pain.

5 HISTORY:
6 Patient is a 63-year-old white male status post fem-pop
7 graft on right and **CABG** in 1982 and now presents with
8 symptoms of **claudication** in left leg. The pain is in
9 the left calf with one block of **ambulation** and he gives
10 no history of pain while resting. Patient states that the pain
11 begins in the calf and migrates to the left foot.
12 Patient also reports sensation loss in the left foot.
13 No history of diabetes, no history of hypertension,
14 chest pain, or myocardial infarction. Patient previously
15 had had **angina** but has had none since surgery and no
16 complaints of **palpitations**.

17 PAST MEDICAL HISTORY:
18 As mentioned above and, in addition, thyroid surgery 12
19 years ago.

20 ALLERGIES:
21 None.

22 MEDICATIONS:
23 None.

24 SOCIAL HISTORY:
25 Smokes two packs a day × 40 years; there is no **ETOH**.

26 FAMILY HISTORY:
27 Positive for coronary artery disease and hypertension.

28 REVIEW OF SYSTEMS:
29 As above.

30 PHYSICAL EXAMINATION AT TIME OF ADMISSION:
31 Remarkable for 2+ regular heart with regular rhythm and
32 rate. Distant heart sound pulses were noted to be 2+
33 in the **carotid**, **radial**, **brachial**, **femoral** on the left
34 and right. No pulse was appreciated in the **popliteal**,
35 **dorsalis pedis** on the right or left, but a palpable
36 right posterior **tibial** was appreciated.

37 Abdomen was soft without masses. Rectal was noted to
38 be **guaiac positive** and not **melanotic**. Question of a
39 prostatic mass 3+ enlargement.

40 LABORATORY DATA AT TIME OF ADMISSION:
41 Electrolytes within normal limits. CBC within normal
42 limits. EKG noted to have a primary A-V block with
43 left anterior hemiblock.

44 Anterior showed a patent right femoral including left
45 **SFA** with three-vessel runoff of **posterior tibialis** to below.

46 HOSPITAL COURSE:
47 Patient was admitted with peripheral vascular disease
48 and question of prostate mass. His hospital course was
49 unremarkable. He had arterial Dopplers performed. The
50 index on the right was noted to be .81 and on the left
51 was noted to be .51. Essentially, this completed the
52 workup for this patient with respect to his claudication.

53 He was discharged on a medication of Trental 400 t.i.d.

54 He was instructed to follow a regular diet and regular
55 activities. Patient was to be scheduled for an
56 outpatient **BE** to rule out malignancy. Patient was also
57 scheduled to have repeat brachial artery index studies.

58 Patient was instructed to follow up in two weeks in the
59 cardiovascular testing clinic.

60 _____
61 Herbert J. Young, MD

62 HJY/urs

63 d: 10/12/—
64 t: 10/12/—   Word Count 422
65 🖽   DSCARMS.2

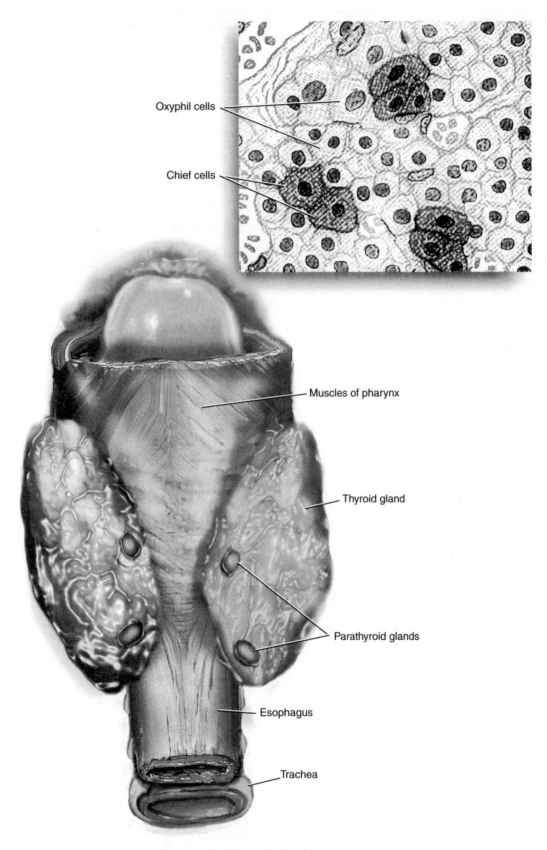

Oxyphil cells

Chief cells

Muscles of pharynx

Thyroid gland

Parathyroid glands

Esophagus

Trachea

Parathyroid glands

dissection	A part or whole of an organism prepared by dissecting.
laryngectomy	Partial or total removal of the larynx by surgery.
thyroid	Resembling a shield; the thyroid gland.
adenoma	A benign epithelial tumor.
hypercalcemic symptoms	Any indication of disease perceived by the patient.
thyroidectomy	Surgical excision of the thyroid gland.
parathyroids	Situated beside the thyroid gland.
afebrile	Without fever.
erythema	Redness of the skin caused by congestion of the capillaries in the lower layers of the skin.
Synthroid	Trademark for a preparation of levothyroxine sodium.

1	PATIENT: Louise Raskin	ADMITTED: 1/20/–
2	CHART #:	DISCHARGED: 1/25/–

1 PATIENT: Louise Raskin ADMITTED: 1/20/–

2 CHART #: DISCHARGED: 1/25/–

3 HISTORY:
4 This is a 58-year-old female with a history of left-
5 sided neck **dissection** and total **laryngectomy** six years
6 ago. She presents now with a **thyroid** mass. She states
7 that a few weeks ago she had a problem swallowing from
8 a fish bone which continued to annoy her after she had it
9 removed. She said that she had a CAT scan done which
10 showed a mass on the thyroid. It was found to be an
11 **adenoma.** She had a feeling of tightness and tickling
12 in the throat. She states that since the operation
13 she has been feeling well and denies weight loss or
14 **hypercalcemic symptoms**.

15 SOCIAL HISTORY:
16 Negative.

17 PAST HISTORY:
18 Negative.

19 PHYSICAL EXAMINATION:
20 A moveable mass on the right side of the thyroid.

21 LABORATORY STUDIES:
22 Within normal limits.

23 HOSPITAL COURSE:
24 The patient was taken to the operating room on the next
25 day where a right **thyroidectomy** was performed with
26 preservation of the **parathyroids.** The patient
27 tolerated the procedure well and remained **afebrile.**

28 Her vital signs remained stable. The flap was clear,
29 dry, and flat on postoperative day number one
30 without **erythema.**

31 The patient continued to do well. The flap remained
32 viable; the incision was clean and closed. She was
33 discharged on postoperative day number four. Followup
34 is with Dr. John Clives.

35 DISCHARGE MEDICATIONS:
36 **Synthroid** 0.1 mg daily.

PATIENT: Louise Raskin
CHART #:
Page 2

37   ACTIVITIES:
38   Ad lib.

39   DIET:
40   Regular.

41   _____

42   Barbara P. Walcott, MD

43   BPW/urs

44   d: 1/25/—
45   t: 1/25/—   Word Count 249
46   DSENDLR.2

biopsy	Excision of living tissue for microscopic examination.
afebrile	Without fever.
ad lib	As desired.

1	PATIENT: Yolanda Guobadia	ADMITTED: 6/5/–	
2	CHART #:	DISCHARGED: 6/8/–	

HISTORY:
This is a 29-year-old severely mentally retarded female
admitted for elective left breast **biopsy** for a large
left breast mass found on routine physical exam.

PAST SURGICAL HISTORY:
Negative.

MEDICATIONS:
Vitamins only.

ALLERGIES:
No known drug allergies.

PHYSICAL EXAMINATION:
A severely contracted female in no apparent distress.
She was **afebrile** with stable vital signs. The patient
had a 2×3 cm irregular mobile mass in the left
breast. The rest of her exam was unremarkable.

HOSPITAL COURSE:
Breast biopsy was performed on June 6 under local
anesthesia. She was brought to the floor
postoperatively with stable vital signs. She was able
to tolerate a diet and void without difficulty. The
patient is being discharged and transferred back to the
Crestwood Developmental Center for followup in the
general surgery clinic.

Medications: None.   Activities: **Ad lib.**

_____
Thomas C. Browne, MD

TCB/urs

d: 6/8/–
t: 6/8/–
⏷

Word Count 160
DSFEMYG.1

metastatic breast carcinoma	Spread of malignancy from primary site (in breast) to other parts of the body through the lymph system or bloodstream.
catheter	A tube passed through the body for evacuating fluids from or injecting fluids into body cavities.
polycystic	Containing many cysts.
myocardial infarction	Condition caused by occlusion of one or more of the coronary arteries.
chemotherapeutic	Of, relating to, or used in chemotherapy.
Inderal	Trademark for a preparation of propranolol hydrochloride.
Capoten	Trademark for a preparation of captopril.
Dilaudid	Trademark for a preparation of hydromorphone, a narcotic analgesic.

1   PATIENT: Eugenia Roman   ADMITTED: 5/18/–

2   CHART #:   DISCHARGED: 5/19/–

3   HISTORY:
4   This is a 48-year-old female with a history of
5   **metastatic breast carcinoma** since 1992 and of severe
6   bone pain for the past two to three years which has
7   worsened recently. The patient presents now for
8   insertion of a MediPort **catheter.**

9   The patient also has a history of **polycystic** kidney
10   disease. She denies lung disease, **myocardial**
11   **infarction,** cardiovascular accident, diabetes,
12   or hypertension.

13   The patient has a long history of multiple
14   **chemotherapeutic** regimens.

15   PAST SURGERY:
16   Right modified radical mastectomy in 1992.

17   ALLERGIES:
18   None.

19   MEDICATIONS:
20   **Inderal** 40 mg daily a.m., **Capoten** and **Dilaudid.**

21   SOCIAL HISTORY:
22   The patient is a nonsmoker, nondrinker, and non-IV
23   drug abuser.

24   PHYSICAL EXAMINATION:
25   Temperature 98.7, pulse 72, respirations 18, blood
26   pressure 120/80. HEENT: Normal. Lungs: Clear.
27   Heart: Regular rhythm, S_1 and S_2.
28   Chest: Mastectomy noted. Abdomen: Soft, nontender,
29   positive bowel sounds. Extremities: edema 1+ in right
30   upper extremity. Neurological: Normal.

31   LABORATORY STUDIES:
32   Within normal limits.

33   HOSPITAL COURSE:
34   The patient underwent the procedure without any
35   complications. She was given three units of packed red
36   blood cells and was deemed stable for discharge the

37 next morning. The MediPort site was clean and
38 functioning well. She was on a regular diet with no new
39 medications. The patient will be followed up as
40 an outpatient.

41   _____

42   Jim Packard, MD

43 JP/urs

44 d: 5/19/—
45 t: 5/19/—   Word Count 233
46   DSFEMER.2

lumpectomy	Surgical excision of only the local lesion in carcinoma of the breast.
axillary lymph node	A rounded body consisting of accumulations of lymphoid tissue in the axillary region (armpit).
gravida	Pregnant woman.
para	Woman who has produced one or more viable offspring.
menarche	Establishment or beginning of the menstrual function.
cholecystectomy	Excision of the gallbladder.
hypertension	Persistently high blood pressure.
Aldomet	Trademark for a preparation of methyldopa, an antihypertensive.
Dyazide	Trademark for a fixed combination preparation of triamterene and hydrochlorothiazide, an antihypertensive.
frozen section	A specimen of tissue that has been quick-frozen, cut by microteme, and stained immediately for rapid diagnosis of possible malignant lesions.
metastatic carcinoma	Spread of malignancy from primary site to other parts of the body through the lymph system or bloodstream.
tomograms	An image of a tissue plane or slice produced by tomography (any of several noninvasive special techniques of roentgenography designed to show detailed images of structures in a selected plane of tissue by blurring images of structures in all other planes).
sacroiliac region	Pertaining to the sacrum and the ilium, or to where these bones meet on both sides of the back.
estrogen	A generic term for estrus-producing compounds; the female sex hormone.

1	PATIENT: Dorothy Sutton	ADMITTED: 4/17/–
2	CHART #:	DISCHARGED: 4/28/–

1   PATIENT: Dorothy Sutton   ADMITTED: 4/17/–

2   CHART #:   DISCHARGED: 4/28/–

3   HISTORY:
4   This 66-year-old woman was admitted with a left breast
5   mass. She presented to the surgical clinic after she
6   noted the mass herself several weeks ago. The patient
7   consented to a **lumpectomy** and **axillary lymph node**
8   dissection.

9   She is **gravida** VI, **para** VI, **menarche** at age 15, first
10   child at 28 years old. The patient used an oral
11   contraceptive for five years in the past and is
12   presently postmenopausal. She has no family history of
13   breast cancer.

14   PAST MEDICAL/SURGICAL HISTORY:
15   **Cholecystectomy** in 1986. **Hypertension** for which she
16   takes **Aldomet** and **Dyazide**.

17   PHYSICAL EXAMINATION:
18   The patient had a large, left upper outer quadrant
19   breast mass as well as matted axillary lymph nodes.
20   The breast mass measured approximately 3×4 cm as well
21   as the axillary mass.

22   HOSPITAL COURSE:
23   The patient was taken to the operating room and had a
24   lumpectomy. A **frozen section** revealed ductal
25   carcinoma; and axillary dissection, which included the
26   highest axillary nodes, was positive for **metastatic**
27   **carcinoma**.

28   Postoperatively, the patient did well; and her Hemovac
29   was removed. She was discharged on April 28, 20– to
30   be followed up in surgery clinic. A bone scan, done
31   while in the hospital, showed abnormal areas of
32   increased activity in the thoracic spine. **Tomograms** of
33   the **sacroiliac region** are recommended for further
34   evaluation. **Estrogen** receptors are pending.

35
36   _____
         Dean Orlando, MD

37   DO/urs

38   d: 4/28/–
39   t: 4/28/–
40   ▄▄

Word Count 241
DSFEMDS.3

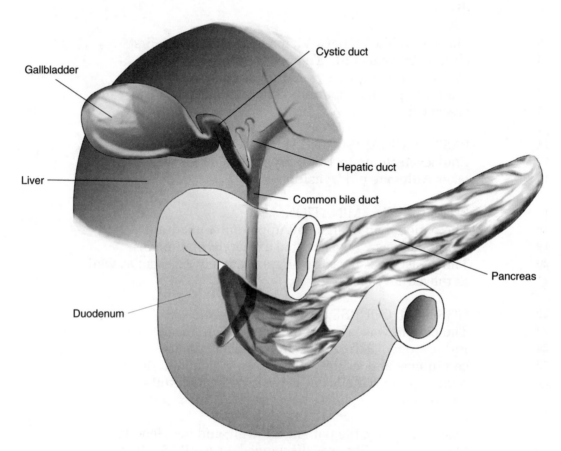

Gallbladder

Cystic duct

Hepatic duct

Common bile duct

Liver

Pancreas

Duodenum

Liver, gallbladder, and pancreas

cholelithiasis	Formation or presence of calculi or bilestones in the gallbladder or common duct.
hepatitis	Inflammation of the liver.
cholecystectomy	Excision of the gallbladder.
analgesics	Drugs that relieve pain.

PATIENT: Julie Wright	ADMITTED: 5/26/–
CHART #:	DISCHARGED: 6/2/–

HISTORY:
This is a 19-year-old female with right upper quadrant
pain, vomiting intermittently after meals, since last
July when she was pregnant. The pain persisted
after meals and during the entire pregnancy. She had a
normal spontaneous vaginal delivery in March of 20–,
and has a normal child.

Since then, she still has persistent pain after meals
in the right upper quadrant which is worse after eating
fatty food. A sonogram was performed at Seaside
Hospital which was significant for **cholelithiasis**. She
had a repeat sonogram at this hospital which showed
cholelithiasis and a normal common bile duct.

PAST MEDICAL HISTORY:
No **hepatitis**, never jaundiced, no intravenous drug use,
and no alcohol use.

PHYSICAL EXAMINATION:
Abdomen was soft, nontender, without masses,
moderately obese, and with striata from pregnancy.

LABORATORY EXAMINATION:
White count 6, hematocrit 37, SMA-6 normal, bilirubin
0.3, alkaline phosphatase 81. Pregnancy, negative.
Ultrasound showed a normal common bile duct, normal with
multiple stones. The impression was cholelithiasis.

HOSPITAL COURSE:
The patient was taken to the operating room on May 27, 20–
where she underwent **cholecystectomy**. Operative
findings were multiple stones in the gallbladder.

Postoperatively, she had a drain which was removed on
postoperative day two. Postoperatively, she had a
fever of 101° for four days which subsequently came
down. Her chest x-ray at that time showed no
infiltrate, and the urine culture showed no growth.

The patient remained afebrile.

PATIENT: Julie Wright
CHART #:
Page 2

37 Upon discharge, a regular diet was prescribed with
38 activity as tolerated.

39 DISCHARGE MEDICATIONS:
40 **Analgesics**.

41 The patient will be followed up in the surgery clinic
42 in one week.

43 _____
44 Clive Wendall, MD

45 CW/urs

46 d: 6/3/—
47 t: 6/4/—   Word Count 289
48 ▰   DSGASJW.1

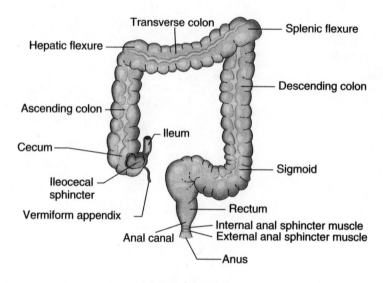

Large intestine

suprapubic	Above the pubis (anterior part of the innominate bone).
hernia	Abnormal protrusion of part of an organ or tissue through the structures normally containing it.
Valsalva's maneuver	Increase of intrathoracic pressure by forcible exhalation against the closed glottis.
heme	The iron-containing nonprotein portion of the hemoglobin molecule wherein the iron is in the ferrous state.
WBC	White blood cell (leukocyte) count.
hemoglobin	An allosteric (pertaining to an effect produced on the biological function of a protein by a compound not directly involved in that function) protein found in erythrocytes that transports molecular oxygen in the blood.
hematocrit	The volume percentage of erythrocytes in whole blood.
electrolyte	A chemical substance which, when dissolved in water or melted, dissociates into electrically charged particles (ions), and thus is capable of conducting an electric current.
amylase	An enzyme that catalyzes the hydrolysis of starch into simpler compounds.
NG tube	Nasogastric tube.
n.p.o.	Nil per os (nothing by mouth).
dilated	Expanded laterally.
hydrated	Addition of water to a substance or tissue.
decompression	The removal of pressure, as from gas in the intestinal tract.
OR	Operating room.
laparotomy	Incision through the flank or, more generally, through any part of the abdominal wall.
lysis	Combining form indicating, in medicine, reduction or relief of.
diverticulosis	Diverticula (sacs or pouches in the walls of a canal or organ) in the colon without inflammation or symptoms.
sigmoid	The sigmoid colon, the distal part of the colon from the level of the iliac crest to the rectum.
transverse colon	Crosswise portion of the large intestine.
angiogram	A radiograph of a blood vessel.

	PATIENT: Margaret Lynch	ADMITTED: 11/3/–

1   PATIENT: Margaret Lynch   ADMITTED: 11/3/–

2   CHART #:   DISCHARGED: 11/26/–

3   HISTORY:
4   This is a 90-year-old female who presented with
5   abdominal pain, crampy and gradual in onset, for the
6   previous two days. She denied nausea, vomiting, fever,
7   or chills. She had had multiple bowel movements for
8   the two days prior to admission. Pain was not radiating.

9   PHYSICAL EXAMINATION:
10   Temperature on admission was 98.0, pulse 102,
11   respirations 18, blood pressure 120/70.

12   She had a softly distended abdomen, very tender,
13   with minimal bowel sounds. She had a healed midline
14   **suprapubic** scar. The patient had a small **hernia**,
15   obvious only on coughing or on **Valsalva's maneuver,** and
16   it was easily reducible. Stool was **heme** positive.

17   LABORATORY STUDIES:
18   **WBC** 13,600; **hemoglobin** 17.7; **hematocrit** 54.9;
19   **electrolytes** normal, **amylase** 61.

20   HOSPITAL COURSE:
21   The patient was admitted with a diagnosis of small
22   bowel obstruction, and an **NG tube** was placed. She was
23   kept **n.p.o**. X-rays showed feces throughout the large
24   bowel in the midabdomen with two **dilated** loops of small
25   bowel with probable air fluid levels.

26   The patient was **hydrated** with **decompression**. On repeat
27   examination, there was no improvement. She was taken
28   to the **OR** and underwent exploratory **laparotomy. Lysis**
29   of adhesions was performed. The patient was noted to
30   have **diverticulosis** of the **sigmoid** and **transverse colon.**

31   An **angiogram** was done, and viability was questionable.

32   The decision was made to take the patient back to the
33   OR for a second look the following day.

34   The patient was taken back to the OR on November 6
35   where exploration revealed a collection of fluid in the
36   bowel and good pulsations.

PATIENT: Margaret Lynch
CHART #:
Page 2

37   Postoperative course was complicated by intermittent
38   noncompliance, poor appetite, and difficulty with bowel
39   movements. The patient was finally discharged on
40   November 26 to be followed up in the surgery clinic.

41   _____

42   Douglas Collins, MD

43   DC/urs

44   d: 11/26/–
45   t: 11/26/–   Word Count 305
46   DSGASML.2

bilaterally	Pertaining to two sides.
pneumothorax	Accumulation of air or gas in the pleural cavity resulting in collapse of the lung on the affected side.
hemidiaphragm	Half of the diaphragm.
intercostal	Between two ribs.
anterior	Situated at or directed toward the front.
axillary	Of or pertaining to the armpit.
Foley	Urinary tract catheter.
exploratory	Investigation or examination for diagnostic purposes.
laparotomy	Incision through the flank, or more generally, through any part of the abdominal wall.
normocephalic	Pertaining to a normal head.
atraumatic	Without injury or damage.
edema	An abnormal accumulation of fluid in intercellular spaces of the body.
laparotomy	Incision through the flank or, more generally, through any part of the abdominal wall.
diaphragmatic	Pertaining to the diaphragm.
p.r.n.	Pro re nata (according to circumstances).

1	PATIENT: Dmitriy Kamenshich	ADMITTED: 6/21/–
2	CHART #:	DISCHARGED: 6/26/–

3 HISTORY:
4 The patient is an 18-year-old male brought to the
5 emergency room after sustaining a gunshot wound of the
6 right upper abdomen posteriorly.

7 The patient, on arrival, had equal breath sounds
8 **bilaterally**, pulse 100/50, heart rate 116,
9 respiratory 18.

10 Chest x-ray showed no **pneumothorax,** but the bullet
11 resting just below the right **hemidiaphragm**.

12 A 40-gauge chest tube was placed in the fifth
13 **intercostal** space **anterior axillary** line which yielded
14 air and scant blood.

15 Urine was heme positive when a **Foley** was passed.
16 Serial abdominal exams revealed increasing diffuse
17 abdominal tenderness, and the patient underwent
18 **exploratory laparotomy**.

19 MEDICATIONS:
20 None.

21 ALLERGIES:
22 None.

23 PAST MEDICAL HISTORY:
24 Medical: None. Surgical: S/P stab wound right thigh
25 in February, 20–, which was left open due to infection.

26 PHYSICAL EXAMINATION:
27 Blood pressure 130/palp, pulse 116, respiration 18.

28 HEENT: **Normocephalic**, **atraumatic**. Lungs: Breath
29 sounds equal bilaterally. Chest tube in right chest.
30 Abdomen: Flat, muscular, grossly nontender,
31 hypoactive bowel sounds. Extremities: Nontender,
32 no **edema**.

33 LABORATORY DATA:
34 Chest x-ray showed chest tube in good position.

HOSPITAL COURSE:
The patient underwent exploratory **laparotomy** at the
time of admission at which time it was noted that he
had a **diaphragmatic** injury and also underwent drainage
of a nonbleeding liver injury.

Postoperatively, the patient's course was unremarkable.

He regained his appetite and was tolerating a regular
diet at the time of discharge.

The patient was on wall suction for his chest tube for
two days at which time it was changed to an underwater
seal. Chest x-ray at that time noted the lung to be
expanded. Subsequently, the chest tube was removed,
and the lung remained expanded.

The patient was discharged with instructions to follow
a regular diet and activity as tolerated. He was to
return to the general surgery clinic on Friday, July 1, 20–,
for staple removal and dressing change. The patient
was instructed to change dressing **p.r.n.** while at home.

_____

Wilbur Hancocks, MD

WH/urs

d: 6/27/–
t: 6/27/–

Word Count 370
DSGASDK.3

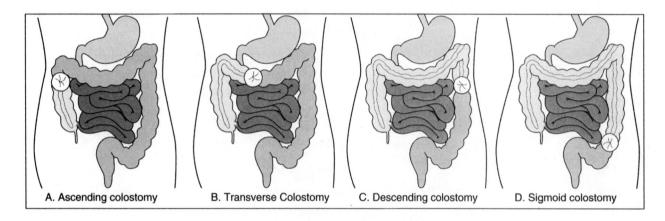

Colostomy sites

colostomy bag	A receptacle worn over the stoma (small, surgically created opening) by a colostomy patient to receive the fecal discharge.
status post	State or condition afterward or following.
transverse colostomy	An artificial opening created in the transverse colon and brought to the surface of the abdomen for the purpose of evacuating the bowels.
sigmoid	The sigmoid colon, the distal part of the colon from the level of the iliac crest to the rectum.
phlegmon	Diffuse inflammation of the soft or connective tissue due to infection.
atherosclerotic heart disease	An extremely common form of arteriosclerosis in which deposits of yellowing plaques containing cholesterol, other lipoid material, and lipophages are formed within the intima of large and medium-sized arteries.
organic brain syndrome	A large group of acute and chronic mental disorders associated with brain damage or impaired cerebral function.
AKA	Above-knee amputation.
COPD	Chronic obstructive pulmonary disease.
AFIB	Atrial fibrillation.
Haldol	Trademark for a preparation of haloperidol, an antipsychotic agent.
anicteric	Without jaundice.

1	PATIENT: Sylvia Hirsch	ADMITTED: 8/2/–
2	CHART #:	DISCHARGED: 8/5/–

HISTORY:
This was one of multiple hospital admissions for this 99-year-old nursing home resident who was transferred here for evaluation of abdominal distension and pain.

The transfer summary relates a 24-hour history of increasing abdominal tenderness and distension with loose bowel movements in the **colostomy bag**. She was **status post** a diverting **transverse colostomy** in June of 20–, for **sigmoid phlegmon,** secondary to tic disease.

PAST MEDICAL HISTORY:
Hypertension, **atherosclerotic heart disease**, **organic brain syndrome**, status post right, hip fracture, status post left **AKA** in March of 20–, status post transverse colostomy, decompensated **COPD,** chronic **AFIB**.

MEDICATION UPON ADMISSION:
The patient is taking Aldomet, Lanoxin, Theo-Dur, zinc oxide, **Haldol** and Kaopectate.

PHYSICAL EXAMINATION:
The patient is a bedridden, elderly female, sleeping comfortably. Temperature 99.4. Vital signs stable. HEENT exam unremarkable. **Anicteric**. Poor respiratory excursion without rales or wheezes. Heart: S1, S2. Abdomen: Softly distended with minimal diffuse tenderness without guarding or rigidity. Bowel sounds present. Rectal: Brown liquid stool, guaiac negative. Extremities: Status post left AKA with a well-healed stump. Right lower extremity, warm, good capillary refill.

LABORATORY DATA ON ADMISSION:
Blood gas of 7.37, 37, 21.5, 87, 96.4% on room air. White count 7.9, hemoglobin and hematocrit 11.9/39.6, platelet count 270,000. Coagulation profile PT/PTT 12.2/23.8.

Abdominal x-ray showed no air fluid levels and no free air under the diaphragm.

REASON FOR ADMISSION:
The patient was admitted for observation and IV antibiotic therapy.

40 HOSPITAL COURSE:
41 The patient was put on IV cefoxitin. A CAT scan of the
42 abdomen with IV and PO contrast was ordered but was not
43 able to be performed secondary to no cooperation from
44 the patient. She recovered from a low-grade fever and
45 was afebrile for 24 hours following discontinuation of
46 her antibiotics.

47 DISPOSITION:
48 The patient was discharged and transferred back to the
49 nursing home. She was tolerating a regular diet and
50 putting out stool and gas through her colostomy.

51 DISCHARGE MEDICATIONS:
52 As per admission, Aldomet, Lanoxin, Theo-Dur, zinc
53 oxide, Haldol, Kaopectate.

54 DISCHARGE DIAGNOSIS:
55 Diverticulosis.

56 _____
57 Ronald T. Ward, MD

58 RTW/urs

59 d: 8/5/—
60 t: 8/5/—   Word Count 358
61 �   DSGASSH.4

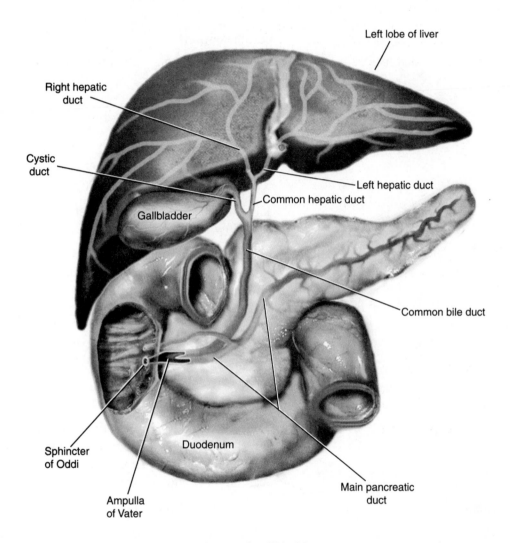

Left lobe of liver

Right hepatic duct

Cystic duct

Left hepatic duct

Common hepatic duct

Gallbladder

Common bile duct

Sphincter of Oddi

Duodenum

Ampulla of Vater

Main pancreatic duct

Liver and gallbladder

anorexia	Loss of appetite.
jaundice	Yellowness of the skin.
anicteric	Without jaundice.
right bundle branch block	A form of heart block involving delay or failure of conduction in the right branch in the Bundle of His.
Q's	Cardiac output.
cholecystitis	Inflammation of the gallbladder.
intrahepatic	Within the liver.
dilatation	Expansion.
calculi	Stones.
cyst	A closed epithelium-lined sac or capsule containing a liquid or semisolid substance.
bilirubin	An orange bile pigment produced by the breakdown of heme and reduction of biliverdin.
AST	Aspartate aminotransferase (an intracellular enzyme involved in amino acid and carbohydrate metabolism).
ERCP	Endoscopic retrograde cholangiopancreatography.
percutaneous catheter	A tubular, flexible instrument passed through the skin for withdrawal of fluids from a body cavity.
cholecystectomy	Excision of gallbladder.
T-tube	Device inserted into biliary duct after removal of gallbladder which allows for drainage and introduction of contrast medium for postoperative cholangiography.
cholangiogram	The film obtained by cholangiography.
duodenum	The first or proximal portion of the small intestine, extending from the pylorus to the jejunum.
drain	Tube for discharge of a morbid matter.
acute	Sharp, severe.
cholelithiasis	Calculi or bilestones in the gallbladder or common duct.
choledocholithiasis	Calculi in the common bile duct.

1	PATIENT: Marilyn Young	ADMITTED: 5/19/–
2	CHART #:	DISCHARGED: 6/6/–

3 HISTORY:
4 This is an 88-year-old female who developed right upper
5 quadrant pain, nausea, **anorexia**, but no vomiting. She
6 had a similar episode in 20– when she was told that
7 she had gallstones. She has no history of **jaundice**.

8 PAST MEDICAL HISTORY:
9 Diabetes, hypertension.

10 MEDICATIONS:
11 Bumex, Tenormin, Naprosyn.

12 PHYSICAL EXAMINATION:
13 Temperature 99.6. Abdomen: Soft, with slight right
14 upper quadrant tenderness. No rebound. No masses.
15 **Anicteric**.

16 EKG revealed atrial enlargement, **right bundle branch**
17 **block**, with **Q's** in 2, 3, and F.

18 SMA-6 showed sodium 151, potassium 5.2, chloride 115,
19 BUN 22, and creatinine 1.9. Glucose 125. White
20 blood cell count 11,700, hemoglobin 11, hematocrit 35.
21 PT 12, PTT 21. Amylase 99. Chest x-ray clear.
22 Abdominal x-ray revealed a large stone in the gallbladder.

23 The patient was admitted with acute **cholecystitis**,
24 dehydration, hypertension, and diabetes.

25 Sonogram revealed a normal liver with mild **intrahepatic**
26 **dilatation** of the gallbladder with **calculi**; common bile
27 duct was a limited evaluation. Cystic duct calculi,
28 and a 9 mm common bile duct were also noted. The left
29 kidney had a **cyst**.

30 Alkaline phosphatase 332, **bilirubin** 7.2 and **AST** 86.

31 HOSPITAL COURSE:
32 The patient was evaluated by Dr. Richard Wagner. The
33 patient was adequately hydrated. An attempt for an
34 **ERCP** for this patient was made, but it was
35 unsuccessful. A **percutaneous catheter** was placed in
36 the common bile duct.

37   On May 21, the patient underwent **cholecystectomy**. A
38   porcelain, calcific gallbladder was removed.

39   Postoperatively, the patient did well. She had a slow,
40   but stable postoperative course. She had some
41   postoperative drainage of bile around the **T-tube**.

42   T-tube **cholangiogram** postoperatively showed a T-tube
43   that had slipped out of the common duct with dye contrast
44   filling the entire common bile duct and flowing freely
45   into the **duodenum**. The T-tube was removed, and a
46   Jackson-Pratt **drain** was also removed. The patient was
47   started on a regular diet and was afebrile. She was
48   discharged to home on June 6.

49   She will be followed up as an outpatient. Diet is
50   regular; activities include light lifting.

51   FINAL DIAGNOSIS:
52   **Acute** cholecystitis, **cholelithiasis**, **choledocholithiasis**.

53   _____
54   Roberta Black, MD

55   RB/urs

56   d: 6/7/—
57   t: 6/8/—   Word Count 356
58   ▰   DSGASMY.5

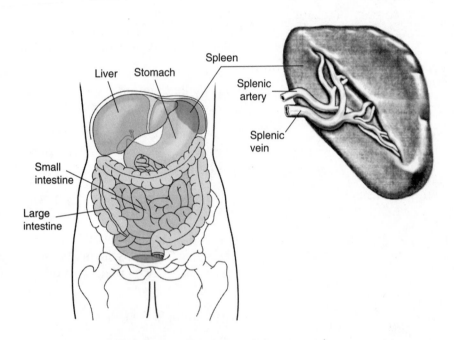

Location of the spleen in the abdominal cavity

peptic ulcer disease	An ulceration of the mucous membrane of the esophagus, stomach, or duodenum, caused by the action of the acid gastric juice.
systolic blood pressure	The greatest force caused by the contraction of the left ventricle of the heart against the walls of the blood vessels.
appendectomy	Excision of the vermiform appendix.
right inguinal hernia	Hernia occurring in the groin.
methadone	A synthetic compound with pharmacologic properties qualitatively similar to those of morphine and heroin.
normocephalic	Normal head attributes.
crepitus	The discharge of flatus from the bowels.
ecchymosis	A hemorrhagic spot, in the skin or mucous membranes, forming a nonelevated, rounded or irregular, blue or purplish patch.
spinous processes	The posterior-most part of a vertebra. This spine projects and serves as a point of attachment for muscles of the back.
blunting costophrenic angle	The space or figure formed by two diverging lines.
hematoma	A localized collection of extravasated (fluid escaping from vessels into surrounding tissue) blood, usually clotted, in an organ, space, or tissue.
splenic	Pertaining to the spleen.
exploratory laparotomy	An abdominal operation for the purpose of investigating or examining for diagnostic purposes.
splenectomy	Excision of the spleen.
Tagamet	Trademark for preparations of cimetidine; used for treatment of peptic ulcer.

1	PATIENT: George DiLorenzo	ADMITTED: 6/5/–
2	CHART #:	DISCHARGED: 6/13/–

3 HISTORY:
4 The patient is a 50-year-old Hispanic male with a
5 history of intravenous drug abuse, alcohol abuse, and
6 **peptic ulcer disease** who was attacked with a baseball
7 bat the afternoon of admission. The patient was struck
8 on the left side of the chest and hip. The patient
9 states he was struck twice. He had no loss of
10 consciousness. The patient complains of
11 left-sided pain.

12 **Systolic blood pressure** in the emergency room was 200.
13 The patient stated that he drank a 12-pack of beer on
14 the day of admission. The patient had nausea and
15 vomited clear fluids.

16 PAST MEDICAL/SURGICAL HISTORY:
17 Intravenous drug abuse. Intravenous cocaine last used
18 one month ago. History of peptic ulcer disease surgery
19 ×2, approximately twenty years ago. Status post
20 **appendectomy**. **Right inguinal hernia** repair. Status
21 post back surgery two years ago.

22 MEDICATIONS:
23 **Methadone**.

24 ALLERGIES:
25 None.

26 SOCIAL HISTORY:
27 Smokes one pack of cigarettes a day. Alcohol abuse.
28 Intravenous drug abuse, cocaine. Denies homosexuality.

29 PHYSICAL EXAMINATION:
30 In moderate distress, unkempt. Head, eyes, ears, nose
31 and throat: **Normocephalic**, atraumatic, neck supple,
32 trachea midline. Respiratory: Decreased breath
33 sounds, left side. Chest: **Crepitus, ecchymosis**, left
34 side of the lower ribs. Heart: Regular rate without
35 murmurs. Abdomen: Soft, positive left upper
36 quadrant pain, without rebound, positive bowel sounds.
37 Back: **Spinous processes** without deformation. Rectal:
38 Normal. Extremities: Left thigh ecchymotic.
39 Neurological examination: Alert, sensory, and motor
40 intact.

PATIENT: George DiLorenzo
CHART #:
Page 2

41 LABORATORY EXAMINATION:
42 White blood cell count 10.3, hematocrit 31.8,
43 hemoglobin 10.7. Electrolytes within normal limits,
44 amylase 96. ABG on admission 7.37, 31, 18, 69 and 93.6.
45 Chest x-ray showed left rib fracture with **blunting**
46 **costophrenic angle**. CT of the abdomen and pelvis
47 showed large **hematoma** on the left.

48 IMPRESSION:
49 Multiple trauma to patient, rule out **splenic** trauma.

50 HOSPITAL COURSE:
51 On the day of admission, the patient went to the
52 operating room and underwent **exploratory laparotomy**
53 with **splenectomy** and tolerated the procedure well.

54 His hospital course was unremarkable. His blood
55 pressure was maintained within normal limits. He was
56 treated with **Tagamet** for his peptic ulcer disease. His
57 chest tube, which had been inserted at the time of
58 admission on the left side, was removed on June 11.
59 The chest remained expanded.

60 At the time of discharge, he was tolerating a regular
61 diet, up and out of bed, and afebrile. The patient was
62 instructed to return to the general surgical clinic on
63 Friday, five days post discharge. He was discharged on
64 a regular diet, given a prescription for Tagamet, and
65 told to resume regular activities as tolerated.

66
67 _____
Paul J. Hazelwood, MD

68 PJH/urs

69 d: 6/13/—
70 t: 6/13/
71 ▣

Word Count 441
DSGASGD.6

DSGENHJ.1	Herbert Jones	Terminology Preview
scrotal		Pertaining to the pouch that contains the testes and accessory organs.
suprapubic		Above the pubic arch.
transilluminating		Inspecting a cavity or organ by passing a light through its walls.
hydrocele		A painless swelling of the scrotum.
elicited		Brought forth, drawn out.
IVP		Intravenous pyelography (a radiograph of the ureter and renal pelvis in which a radiopaque material is administered through a vein).
benign		Not malignant.
hematocele		A blood cyst.
marsupialized		Conversion of a closed cavity into an open pouch by incising it and suturing the edges of its wall to the edges of the wound.
scrotum		Pouch that contains the testes and accessory organs.
penis		External male organ of urination and copulation.
edema		A local or generalized condition in which the body tissues contain an excessive amount of tissue fluid.
prepuce		A cutaneous fold over the glans penis.
Geocillin		Trade name for carbenicillin indanyl sodium.
tetracycline		A member of the tetracycline group of broad-spectrum antibiotics having similar pharmacological activity.

PUNCTUATION REFERENCES

Lines 4, 9	hyphens—compound modifier, Rule 1
Line 12	commas—series, Rule 1
Line 14	commas—apposition, Rule 7
Line 15	comma—parenthetical, Rule 10
Line 19	comma—two-adjective modifiers, Rule 2

Line 22	comma—date and year, Rule 4
Lines 23, 26	commas—conjunction, Rule 3
Line 28	apostrophe—singular possessive, Rule 1
Line 28	commas—nonrestrictive clause, Rule 8
Line 29	comma—introductory word, Rule 7
Line 30	apostrophe—singular possessive, Rule 1
Lines 31, 33	commas—conjunction, Rule 3

1	PATIENT: Herbert Jones
2	CHART #:

	ADMITTED: 10/29/–
	DISCHARGED: 11/5/–

3 HISTORY:
4 The patient was admitted with a six-month history of
5 right **scrotal** swelling. He had been treated for
6 hypertension but no longer takes pills. No other
7 medical or surgical history was available.

8 PHYSICAL EXAMINATION:
9 Examination revealed a 62-year-old apparently healthy
10 male not complaining of any specific thing. Blood
11 pressure was stable at 140/80. Abdomen was soft with
12 no masses, no areas of tenderness, no lumbar or
13 **suprapubic** masses or tenderness. Genitalia showed the
14 right scrotum, fist size, high up against the pubic
15 bone, **transilluminating**. The impression was a right
16 **hydrocele**.

17 No impulse of coughing was **elicited**.

18 **IVP** showed a normal upper tract. Rectal examination
19 showed a small, soft **benign** prostatic mass.

20 HOSPITAL COURSE:
21 The patient was taken to the operating room on
22 October 30, 20–, at which time a right **hematocele** was
23 found. This was excised, and the edges were
24 **marsupialized** back of the cord. Drains were left in
25 the **scrotum** and removed on the second postoperative
26 day. The scrotal swelling was moderate, but there was
27 a lot of deformity to the **penis** with **edema** of the **prepuce**.

28 The patient's temperature, which rose to 102° at times,
29 was finally controlled with antibiotics. Presently,
30 the swelling is down. The patient's temperature is
31 down, and the tenderness is gone. The patient is now
32 being discharged for office followup. The patient had
33 been given **Geocillin** during this hospital stay, and now
34 he will be placed on **tetracycline** 500 mg twice a day.

35 FINAL DIAGNOSIS: Right hematocele.

36 _____
37 Maria A. Sidoti, MD

38 MAS/urs

39 d: 11/6/–
40 t: 11/6/–
41 📼

Word Count 149
DSGENHJ.1

appendectomy	Excision of the vermiform appendix.
CVA	Costovertebral (pertaining to a rib and a vertebra) angle.
IVP	Intravenous pylelogram (a radiograph of the ureter and renal pelvis in which a radiopaque material is administered through a vein).
pyelovenous extravasation	A discharge or escape, as of blood, from a vessel (renal veins) into the tissues (renal pelvis).
distal	Farthest from the center.
ureter	The fibromuscular tube, 16 to 18 inches long, through which the urine passes from the kidney to the bladder.
sedated	Calmed down, quieted, tranquilized.
asymptomatic	Showing no symptoms.
KUB	A plain film of the abdomen, providing information about abdominal organs including the kidneys, ureters, and bladder.
leiomyomatous	Related to a fibroma (consisting principally of smooth muscle tissue).
fibroid	Colloquial term for fibroma (a fibrous, encapsulated connective tissue tumor).
gynecologist	Physician specialist in gynecology.

1	PATIENT: Etta Farthings	ADMITTED: 4/7/–
2	CHART #:	DISCHARGED: 4/9/–

HISTORY:
This 68-year-old woman was admitted through the
emergency room with an acute onset of left flank and
left abdominal pain starting about 3 a.m. on the day of
admission. She had had no previous episodes of similar
pain. There was nausea and vomiting associated with
the present symptoms. The patient had an **appendectomy**
in 20–.

PHYSICAL EXAMINATION:
Blood pressure: 190/105. Temperature: Normal.
Abdomen: Slightly distended. Some moderate left lower
quadrant tenderness and mild left **CVA** tenderness.
Chest: Lungs, clear. Heart: Regular rhythm.
Neck: Supple.

LABORATORY DATA:
Urinalysis 15–20 RBCs per high-powered field. CBC: WBC
7560, 80.9 neutrophils, 13.4% lymphs.
SMA-12 glucose: 200. Creatinine: 1.3. BUN: 27.
Remainder of SMA-12: Normal.
Chest x-ray: Negative. **IVP**: Slight delay in
excretion on the left. Some **pyelovenous extravasation**.
Small stone at the **distal ureter** with colonization of
the left ureter down to the stone.

HOSPITAL COURSE:
The patient was **sedated** and kept on IV fluids. She
became **asymptomatic** on the day following admission and
remained so. **KUB** revealed calculus changing position
from the area of the distal left ureter down into the
bladder. On the x-ray some calcific densities
overlying the sacrum were felt to be secondary to a
leiomyomatous uterus. The patient has a history of
a **fibroid**.

At the time of discharge, the patient was asymptomatic.
KUB again showed free-floating stone in the bladder.
A pelvic sonogram was ordered; however, because of
equipment problems, it was not done. The patient was,
therefore, discharged and told to strain urines. She
will make an appointment with her **gynecologist** for

PATIENT: Etta Farthings
CHART #:
Page 2

41   further followup of possible pelvic mass. She will
42   also see Dr. Fred Elliott for followup in about two weeks.

43

44   James D. Howell, MD

45   JDH/urs

46   d: 4/10/—
47   t: 4/11/—   Word Count 312
48   ▰▰   DSGENEF.2

groin	The junction between the abdomen and thigh.
testicular	Pertaining to the testis.
peptic ulcer disease	An ulceration of the mucous membrane of the esophagus, stomach, or duodenum.
ecchymosis	Hemorrhagic spot, in the skin or mucous membranes, forming a nonelevated, rounded or irregular, blue or purplish patch.
inguinal area	Pertaining to the groin area.
hemoglobin	An allosteric protein found in erythrocytes that transports molecular oxygen in the blood.
hematocrit	The volume percentage of erythrocytes in whole blood.
UA	Urinalysis.
intravenous	Within a vein.
epididymis	An elongated, cordlike structure along the posterior border of the testis.
epididymitis	Inflammation of the epididymis.
scrotal hematoma	A localized collection of extravasated blood in the scrotum.
afebrile	Without fever.
Vibramycin	Trademark for preparations of doxycycline; a tetracycline antibiotic.
GU	Genitourinary.

PATIENT: Cliff Morton	ADMITTED: 5/7/–
CHART #:	DISCHARGED: 5/11/–

HISTORY:
The patient is a 34-year-old black male who stated he was assaulted on the evening of admission by several men. The patient stated he was struck with an object in the right side of the back and in the **groin.** He came to the emergency room complaining of right **testicular** pain which radiated to the groin.

The patient denied burning, frequency, or urgency on urination. He denied urinary tract symptoms prior to this incident. He denied loss of consciousness or head trauma.

PAST MEDICAL HISTORY:
Significant only for **peptic ulcer disease,** status post upper GI bleed which was treated medically in 20–.

PAST SURGICAL HISTORY:
None.

MEDICATIONS:
Denied.

ALLERGIES:
Denied.

SOCIAL HISTORY:
Patient has smoked one pack of cigarettes per day for several years. He uses alcohol heavily. He has a past history of IV drug abuse but has not used IV drugs for four years prior to this admission.

PHYSICAL EXAMINATION:
Fair amount of swelling in the right scrotal sac. Small amount of **ecchymosis** bilaterally. Right testicle somewhat tender to palpation and tender in the right **inguinal area.** Prostate smooth but extremely tender and mildly enlarged. Remainder of physical exam unremarkable.

LABORATORY DATA:
Significant for WBC 11.8. **Hemoglobin** and **hematocrit** within normal limits, platelets, normal.

38 Chemistries: Within normal limits. **UA:** Innumerable
39 white blood cells in urine with only 0 to 3 red cells.

40 HOSPITAL COURSE:
41 The patient was admitted to the urological services of
42 Dr. Barry Gregson. He was placed on **intravenous** antibiotics,
43 and a testicular nuclear medicine scan was obtained.
44 The scan revealed normal blood flow to both testicles.
45 There was increased uptake in the **epididymis** of the
46 affected testicle, interpreted as traumatic
47 **epididymitis.** This was followed up by a testicular
48 sonogram which revealed a small **scrotal hematoma.** No
49 evidence of a ruptured testicle was found.

50 The patient was maintained on intravenous antibiotics
51 and scrotal support and soaks. He has improved
52 significantly over the course of his admission. He has
53 become and remained **afebrile.** His white count
54 decreased. He is now being discharged in a much
55 improved condition. He will be given a prescription
56 for **Vibramycin** and will be on a regular diet with activities
57 as tolerated with no strenuous activity. He will
58 follow up in **GU** clinic in one week.

59
60 _____
    Ronald Ford, MD

61 RF/urs

62 d: 5/12/—
63 t: 5/12/—   Word Count 416
64   DSGENCM.3

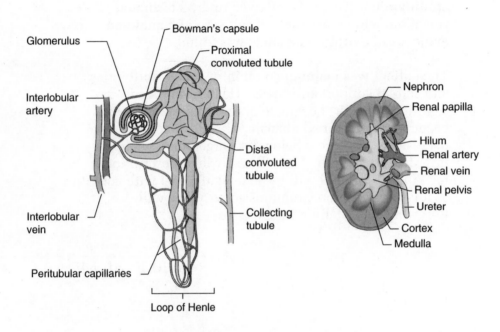

Nephron; cross section of kidney

renal calculus	Kidney stone.
dysuria	Painful or difficult urination.
anorexia	Lack or loss of appetite for food.
hypertension	Persistently high blood pressure.
Lasix	Trademark for preparation of furosemide, a diuretic (an agent that increases urine secretion).
thyroidectomy	Surgical excision of the thyroid gland.
hysterectomy	Surgical removal of the uterus.
defervesced	Return to normal body temperature following a fever.
E. coli	*Escherichia coli.*
lithotripsy	The crushing of calculi in the bladder, urethra, kidney, or gallbladder.

1	PATIENT: Yoshie Takahashi	ADMITTED: 2/28/–
2	CHART #:	DISCHARGED: 3/9/–

1   PATIENT: Yoshie Takahashi   ADMITTED: 2/28/–

2   CHART #:   DISCHARGED: 3/9/–

3   HISTORY:
4   The patient is a 70-year-old female with a one-day
5   history of fever, chills, and right flank pain. She
6   has no history of **renal calculus** but has had frequent
7   urinary tract infections. She has **dysuria** at present.
8   The patient denies nausea, vomiting, **anorexia,** or
9   abdominal pain.

10   PAST MEDICAL HISTORY:
11   Significant for **hypertension.** She denies diabetes,
12   coronary artery disease, or other medical problems.

13   MEDICATIONS:
14   **Lasix** 20 mg by mouth each day.

15   PAST SURGICAL HISTORY
16   Total **thyroidectomy** in 20– and a radical **hysterectomy**
17   ten years prior to admission.

18   ALLERGIES:
19   No known allergies.

20   SOCIAL HISTORY:
21   The patient has smoked one to two packs of cigarettes
22   per day for fifty years. She drinks alcohol
23   occasionally. The patient denies intravenous
24   drug abuse.

25   PHYSICAL EXAMINATION:
26   On admission, the physical examination is remarkable
27   for an elderly female in mild distress.

28   Temperature, 103° on admission and at the time of
29   physical examination, 99.8° after Tylenol. Blood
30   pressure 110/70, respirations 20.

31   The patient is awake and alert and oriented ×3,
32   well developed, and well nourished. Heart has a regular
33   rhythm with no murmurs. Head, eyes, ears, nose, and
34   throat are within normal limits. Neck is supple with
35   no masses. Lungs are clear bilaterally.

36   There is marked right costovertebral angle tenderness.

37 Abdomen is soft and nontender, no masses, normoactive
38 bowel sounds. Rectal is heme negative; no masses
39 are present.

40 Extremities: Without edema.

41 Neurological: The patient is intact.

42 LABORATORY EXAMINATION:
43 On admission, white cell count 10.6, hematocrit 39,
44 hemoglobin 12.5. SMA-6 within normal limits.

45 Urinalysis significant for 3+ protein hemoglobin and 10
46 to 12 RBC greater than 200 WBC in the field. The rest
47 of the studies were within normal limits.

48 Abdominal x-ray revealed a large stone in the right
49 renal pelvis. Chest x-ray, unremarkable.
50 EKG, unremarkable.

51 HOSPITAL COURSE:
52 The patient was admitted to the urological service of
53 Dr. Robert Ronard and was placed on intravenous Ancef
54 after blood and urine cultures had been taken. The
55 patient rapidly **defervesced**. Urine cultures grew
56 *E. coli* sensitive to Ancef.

57 The patient had a very good clinical response and was
58 maintained on intravenous Ancef as per the infectious disease
59 consult with Dr. Leonard Logger.

60 The patient has done very well and is currently pain-
61 free and afebrile. She has completed a nine-day course
62 of IV antibiotics and is now discharged in a much
63 improved condition with a prescription for Keflex by
64 mouth. She will have followup with Dr. Ronard in the
65 office. Dr. Ronard will arrange for **lithotripsy** of the
66 stone. The patient is to follow a regular diet, to
67 drink plenty of fluids to keep herself well hydrated,
68 and to avoid strenuous activity.

69 _____
70 Michael James Boyle, MD

71 MJB/urs

72 d: 3/9/—
73 t: 3/9/—   Word Count 456
74 🔖   DSGENYT.4

DSMUSDL.2	David Lopez	Terminology Preview
scapula		The large, flat triangular bone that forms the posterior part of the shoulder (shoulder blade).
intercostal space		Space between two ribs.
dyspnea		Difficult, painful breathing.
hemoptysis		Coughing and spitting of blood as a result of bleeding from any part of the respiratory tract.
SMA-6		Sequential Multiple Analysis—six different serum tests.
pneumothorax		Accumulation of air or gas in the pleural cavity, resulting in collapse of the lung on the affected side.
hemothorax		Collection of blood in the pleural cavity.

PUNCTUATION REFERENCES

Line 4	hyphens—compound modifier, Rule 1
Line 6	commas—parenthetical, Rule 10
Line 8	commas—parenthetical, Rule 10
Line 12	comma—introductory phrase, Rule 7
Lines 12, 13	commas—series, Rule 1
Line 13	hyphen—certain adjective forms, Rule 4
Line 24	comma—parenthetical, Rule 10
Line 28	comma—for separation (like city and state), Rule 4
Lines 36, 37	commas—series, Rule 1

1	PATIENT: David Lopez	ADMITTED: 5/16/–
2	CHART #:	DISCHARGED: 5/17/

3 HISTORY:
4 The patient is a 17-year-old male admitted through the
5 emergency room presenting shortly after having been
6 stabbed one time. The stab wound, by knife, is in the
7 right posterior chest at the level of the tip of the
8 **scapula**, right seventh **intercostal space**, approximately
9 2 cm off the posterior midline. The wound was said to
10 be approximately 4 cm in length and 1 to 2-1/2 inches
11 in width.

12 At the time of admission, the patient denied **dyspnea**,
13 **hemoptysis**, dizziness, light-headedness, nausea
14 or vomiting.

15 MEDICATIONS:
16 None.

17 PAST MEDICAL HISTORY:
18 Unremarkable.

19 PAST SURGICAL HISTORY:
20 Gunshot wound requiring admission in February, 20–.

21 PHYSICAL EXAMINATION:
22 The patient was noted to have a knife wound
23 approximately 4 cm in length and 2 inches in width at
24 the right seventh intercostal inner space, 2 cm from
25 the tip of the scapula. Examination was
26 otherwise unremarkable.

27 LABORATORY DATA:
28 Hemoglobin 14.5, hematocrit 44.0. **SMA**-6 within normal
29 limits. Chest x-ray was without **pneumothorax**.

30 HOSPITAL COURSE:
31 The patient was kept under observation for 24 hours.
32 Repeat chest x-ray was performed on May 17. No change
33 was noted from his admission chest x-ray. No
34 **pneumothorax** or **hemothorax** was noted.

35 The patient was discharged on May 17 with no
36 medications, on a regular diet, activities as

PATIENT: David Lopez
CHART #:
Page 2

37   tolerated, and plans for followup in general surgery
38   clinic on May 20.

39   _____
40   Kevin Youngblood, MD

41   KY/urs

42   d: 5/18/—
43   t: 5/18/—   Word Count 243
44   DSMUSDL.2

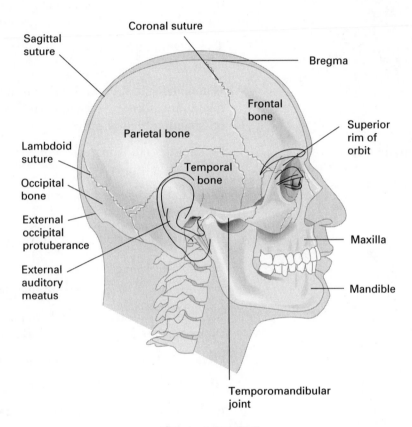

Bones of the skull

status post	State or condition afterward or following.
ambulate	Walk.
ER	Emergency room.
tympanic membranes	Thin layers of tissue covering the middle ear or tympanic cavity.
hematotympanum	Hemorrhage into the middle ear.
subconjunctival hemorrhage	Escape of blood from a ruptured vessel into the conjunctiva (mucous membranes lining the eyelids) reflected onto the eyeball.
mucosal edema	The accumulation of excess fluid in the mucous membranes.
ecchymosis	A hemorrhagic spot, in the skin or mucous membrane, forming a nonelevated, rounded or irregular, blue or purplish patch.
temporomaxillary juncture	Pertaining to the juncture of the temporal bone and maxilla (upper jaw).
zygomatic fracture	Break in the zygomatic bone (bone on either side of the face below the eye).
mandibular	Pertaining to the bone of the lower jaw.
tripod fracture	Fracture in three places.
PT, PTT	Prothrombin time, partial thromboplastin time.
costophrenic angle	The lateral, inferior corner of the pulmonary cavity bordered by the ribs and diaphragm.
tri-malar fracture	Pertaining to triple fracture of cheekbones.
ORIF	Open reduction, internal fixation.
condyle	A rounded projection on a bone, usually for articulation with another bone.
p.o.	By mouth.

1	PATIENT: Frank Aaron	ADMITTED: 9/23/–
2	CHART #:	DISCHARGED: 10/15/–

3 HISTORY:
4 This is a 66-year-old male **status post** fracture trauma
5 one day prior to admission.

6 The patient states that he was beaten with an unknown
7 object while intoxicated. He reports loss of
8 consciousness for a few minutes. However, he awakened
9 and was able to **ambulate** to the police station where he
10 reported the incident.

11 The patient came to the emergency room with complaints
12 of facial pain and swelling. He has been unable to
13 chew food and his left eye is swollen and closed. The
14 patient last drank two to three beers just prior to
15 coming to the **ER** and last ate at 2 p.m. yesterday.

16 He denied shortness of breath, chest pain, or visual-
17 hearing changes.

18 PAST MEDICAL HISTORY:
19 No diabetes, no hypertension, no peptic ulcer disease.

20 PAST SURGERY:
21 Hernia repair, right knee surgery.

22 ALLERGIES:
23 None.

24 SOCIAL HISTORY:
25 Alcohol abuse, no IV drug abuse.

26 PHYSICAL EXAMINATION:
27 Elderly male, awake, alert, and dressed neatly in moderate
28 distress. HEENT: Skull without evidence of fractures.
29 **Tympanic membranes** clean. No **hematotympanum**.
30 Eyes: Positive left **subconjunctival hemorrhage**, left
31 lid closed, slight limitation of left upward gaze.
32 Nose: No fractures. Throat: Posterior pharynx clean.
33 Mouth: **Mucosal edema** and **ecchymosis**. No opening of
34 intra-oral wounds or continuous fractures. Positive
35 dentures upper and lower.

36 Face: Severe left-sided edema and ecchymosis, left
37 **temporomaxillary juncture** tenderness, left infra-
38 orbital rim tender with palpable step-off. Left
39 palpable **zygomatic fracture**, lateral one-third and left
40 **mandibular** tender laterally.

41 Heart: Regular rhythm. Lungs: Clear bilaterally.
42 Chest: With ecchymosis, extending to the left nipple.
43 Abdomen: Soft, nondistended, no masses, no
44 organomegaly. Extremities: Positive pulses
45 throughout.

46 X-ray: Left **tripod fracture**, left zygomatic fracture,
47 left mandibulum, old fracture. No nasal fractures.
48 Left infra-orbital rim fracture, left maxillary
49 wall fracture.

50 LABORATORY STUDIES:
51 White count 9400, hematocrit 45.9, hemoglobin 15.1,
52 platelet count 298,000. Electrolytes: Normal.
53 **PT**, **PTT**: Normal. EKG: Normal sinus rhythm.
54 Chest x-ray: Old rib fracture on the left, normal air
55 density, slight blunting of the left **costophrenic angle**.

56 HOSPITAL COURSE:
57 The patient was admitted and, on the second hospital
58 day, he underwent facial wound reconstruction ×3, open
59 reduction, internal fixation of the left **tri-malar**
60 **fracture**, exploration of left orbital floor, **ORIF**, left
61 mandibular **condyle** and placement of intramaxillary
62 fixation to upper and lower prefixed dental plates and
63 anterior maxillary fixation.

64 The patient tolerated the procedure well. He was kept
65 on Ancef and Oxacillin.

66 The patient did well postoperatively. Sutures were
67 removed. The swelling of his face subsided. He was
68 discontinued on antibiotics and remained afebrile.
69 At the time of discharge, he was up and out of bed. He
70 was able to tolerate **p.o.** fluids through a straw. He
71 had a liquefied regular diet which he tolerated well.
72 He was discharged on October 15 and placed on a

73 liquefied regular diet and instructed to follow up with
74 ophthalmology, general surgery, maxilla-facial surgery
75 and plastic surgery clinics.

76 _____
77   Peter Ashford, MD

78 PA/urs

79 d: 10/16/—
80 t: 10/16/—   Word Count 510
81   DSMUSFA.3

lumbar laminectomy	Surgical excision of a vertebral posterior arch in the lumbar region of the spine.
radiating	Spreading from a common center.
CAT	Computed axial tomography.
myelogram	Roentgenogram of the spinal canal after injection of radiopaque dye.
herniated	Protruding like a hernia.
nucleus pulposus	The soft part of the intervertebral disk.

| 1 | PATIENT: Valerie Sullivan | ADMITTED: 4/25/– |
| 2 | CHART #: | DISCHARGED: 4/25/– |

HISTORY:
This is a 47-year-old female who was admitted for an elective **lumbar laminectomy** this morning. The patient has a history of low back pain, **radiating** down the right lower extremity for the past year.

A **CAT** scan and **myelogram** reveal a **herniated nucleus pulposus** at L4 and L5.

On questioning, the patient admitted to aspirin use for the past four days. She was informed that her operation might be cancelled if further tests showed abnormal platelet aggregation.

The patient did have an abnormal platelet aggregation profile; and, therefore, she is being discharged today, April 25, 20–, for elective readmission in the future. The patient is going to be given a prescription for Fioricet for tension headache.

_____

Collin Webster, MD

CW/urs

d: 4/25/–
t: 4/25/–

Word Count 148
DSNERVS.1

lumbar myelogram	Roentgenogram of the lumbar region (five bones of the spinal column between the sacrum and thoracic vertebrae) after injection of radiopaque dye.
CT	Computerized tomography.
Decadron	Trademark for preparations of dexamethasone, an anti-inflammatory adrenocortical steroid.
q.6h.	Daily, every six hours.
Diabinese	Trademark for chlorpropamide, an oral hypoglycemic (pertaining to a deficiency of blood sugar) drug.
Isordil	Trademark for a preparation of isosorbide, a coronary vasodilator.
Persantine	Trademark for preparations of dipyridamole, a coronary vasodilator.
insulin	A double-chain protein hormone formed from proinsulin in the beta cells of the pancreatic islets of Langerhans.
E. coli (Escherichia coli)	A strain of bacteria common to the alimentary canal of humans and animals.
catheterization	Passage of a catheter (tube) into a body channel or cavity for evacuation of fluid.
OR	Operating room.
laminectomy	Surgical excision of a vertebral posterior arch of the spine.
intradural	Within or enclosed by the dura mater (the outer membrane covering the spinal cord).
extramedullary	Situated outside the marrow or inner portion of the spinal cord.
meningioma	A slow-growing tumor that originates in the arachnoidal tissue (one of the three membranes (middle membrane) investing the spinal cord and brain).
PO	Postoperative.
ICU	Intensive care unit.
extubated	Removal of a previously inserted tube from an organ orifice or other body structure.
p.o.	By mouth.
q.d.	Every day.
t.i.d.	Three times a day.
MOM	Milk of Magnesia.
ADA	American Diabetes Association.

1	PATIENT: Irena Svetsky	ADMITTED: 4/15/–
2	CHART #:	DISCHARGED: 4/28/–

3 HISTORY:
4 This patient is a 76-year-old Russian-speaking woman,
5 electively admitted to the hospital surgery service
6 for a **lumbar myelogram**.

7 The patient complained of four to six months of an
8 aggressive onset of loss of sensation and strength of
9 the muscles in both lower extremities with the right
10 loss greater than the left.

11 A **CT** myelogram performed on April 14 revealed a
12 complete block at the T4 level. The patient was placed
13 on **Decadron** 4 mgs **q.6h.** Her preadmission medications,
14 **Diabinese**, **Isordil**, and **Persantine** were discontinued
15 preadmission.

16 The patient's fasting blood sugar levels were greater
17 than 240, and regular **insulin** coverage was instituted.
18 *Escherichia coli* were grown from urine in routine
19 preoperative lab tests. The *E. coli* cells were
20 sensitive to ampicillin, and the patient was started on
21 this medication. The patient required **catheterization**
22 for urinary retention preoperatively.

23 HOSPITAL COURSE:
24 The patient went to the **OR** on April 19 for a T2–T3,
25 T4–T5 **laminectomy** and removal of a partially calcified
26 well-circumscribed **intradural**, **extramedullary** lesion.
27 The pathology report was suspicious for **meningioma**.
28 **PO** the patient was brought to the neurosurgery **ICU** and
29 was **extubated** on the following day. The glucose
30 was well controlled, and the patient was transferred to the
31 floor on PO day two. Rehabilitation was instituted
32 with Russian-speaking doctor, Dr. Igor Slovetsky. On PO day
33 four, the patient was restarted on Diabinese, and she
34 had the boots removed on PO day six.

35 The patient is being discharged on April 28, 20–, from
36 general surgery service and will be transferred to
37 rehabilitation service.

38 DIAGNOSIS:
39 Spinal cord meningioma.

PATIENT: Irena Svetsky
CHART #:
Page 2

40   CONDITION:
41   Stable and doing very well.

42   MEDICATIONS TRANSFER:
43   Diabinese 250 mg **p.o., q.d.,** Isordil 5 mg po **t.i.d.,** Colace
44   100 mg po tid, **MOM**, and Motrin.

45   Activity as per Rehab. Diet with 1800-calorie **ADA** diet.

46   _____

47   Lillian Campbell, MD

48   LC/urs

49   d: 4/28/–
50   t: 4/28/–   Word Count 317
51   DSNERIS.2

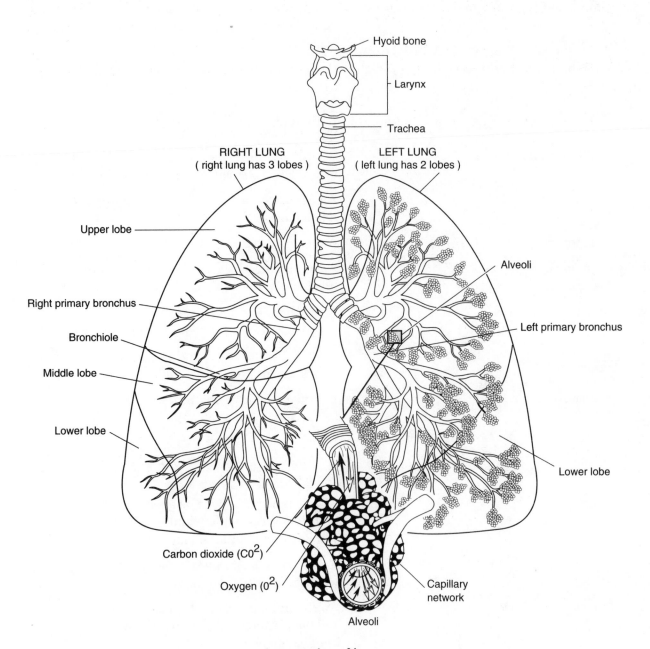

Hyoid bone

Larynx

Trachea

RIGHT LUNG
(right lung has 3 lobes)

LEFT LUNG
(left lung has 2 lobes)

Upper lobe

Alveoli

Right primary bronchus

Left primary bronchus

Bronchiole

Middle lobe

Lower lobe

Lower lobe

Carbon dioxide (CO_2)

Oxygen (O_2)

Capillary
network

Alveoli

Cross section of lungs

tuberculosis	An infectious, inflammatory, reportable disease that is chronic in nature and commonly affects the lungs.
chronic obstructive pulmonary disease	A functional category designating a chronic condition of persistent obstruction of bronchial air flow.
aspiration pneumonia	Pneumonia after inhaling foreign matter into the lungs.
infiltrate	To penetrate the interstices of a tissue or substance.
acid-fast bacilli	Bacilli not readily decolorized by acids or other means when stained.
isoniazid	An antibacterial used principally in treating tuberculosis.
ethambutol	A tuberculostatic agent.
streptomycin	An antibiotic substance, used chiefly in the treatment of tuberculosis.
rifampin	A semisynthetic antibacterial derived from rifamycin SV, used in treatment of pulmonary tuberculosis.
LFT	Low-frequency tetanic (stimulation).
clindamycin	A semisynthetic antibiotic derivative of lincomycin, used as an antibacterial and antiparasitic agent.
anemic	Pertaining to anemia (abnormal reduction of red blood cells).
central line	A venous access device inserted into and kept in the vein in order to maintain a route for administering fluids and medicines.
basilar pneumothorax	A collection of air or gas in the pleural cavity which is of primary importance.
bronchopleural fistula	An abnormal passage between the bronchus and the pleura, resulting from abscesses or inflammation.
purulent	Containing or forming pus.
AFB	Acid-fast bacillus.
parenchyma	The essential or functional elements of an organ in contradistinction to its framework.

DSRESSS.1	Stanley Staples	Terminology Preview
pleural		Pertaining to the serous membrane that enfolds both lungs and is reflected upon the walls of the thorax and diaphragm.
speciation		The evolutionary formation of new species.
MTB		*Mycobacterium tuberculosis.*
thoracotomy		Incision of the chest wall.
necrotic		Related to death of a portion of tissue.
bifurcation		A division into two branches.
pneumonectomy		Excision of lung tissue, of an entire lung, or less, or of a single lobe.

PUNCTUATION REFERENCES

Line 4	hyphen—compound modifier, Rule 1
Line 9	apostrophe—singular possessive, Rule 1
Line 11	comma—conjunction, Rule 3
Line 12	hyphen—compound modifier, Rule 1
Line 12	semicolon—second independent clause contains series commas
Line 13	commas—series, Rule 1
Line 18	comma—introductory phrase, Rule 7
Line 19	comma—conjunction, Rule 3
Line 22	comma—conjunction, Rule 3
Line 25	comma—introductory phrase, Rule 7
Lines 27, 31	comma—conjunction, Rule 3
Line 32	comma—introductory word, Rule 7
Line 37	comma—introductory phrase, Rule 7
Line 47	comma—introductory word, Rule 7
Line 53	semicolon—second independent clause contains commas
Line 53	commas—parenthetical, Rule 10

1	PATIENT: Stanley Staples
2	CHART #:

ADMITTED: 2/1/–

DISCHARGED: 4/20/–

3   HISTORY:
4   Mr. Staples is a 38-year-old male with a history of IV
5   drug abuse and **tuberculosis** as well as **chronic**
6   **obstructive pulmonary disease** and hypertension. He was
7   admitted for probable **aspiration pneumonia**.

8   HOSPITAL COURSE:
9   The patient's hospital course has been long and
10   complicated. His admission chest x-ray revealed a left
11   lung **infiltrate**, and he was placed on penicillin.
12   Sputum was positive for **acid-fast bacilli;** and he was
13   also placed on **isoniazid, ethambutol,** and **streptomycin**.
14   The **rifampin** was discontinued because of increasing **LFT**.

15   The patient continued to have spiking temperatures in
16   spite of treatment and was put on **clindamycin**. He was
17   also found to be **anemic** with a hematocrit of 24.
18   Because of his IV drug abuse, he had an access problem.
19   A **central line** was attempted on February 8, and this
20   led to a left **basilar pneumothorax**.

21   A chest tube was placed on February 9 with minimal
22   resolution of the pneumothorax, but a **bronchopleural**
23   **fistula** was created producing **purulent** drainage. This
24   discharge was found to be positive for **AFB**. By chest
25   x-ray and CAT scan, the chest tube was seen to be in
26   the lung **parenchyma**.

27   On February 12 this chest tube was pulled, and a new
28   one was placed in the **pleural** space. This tube
29   continued to drain greater than 50 cc of greenish fluid
30   per day.

31   The fluid was sent to the lab for AFB weekly, and the
32   results were found to be negative. However, the
33   bronchopleural fistula remained. The weekly chest
34   x-ray showed no change in the pneumothorax.
35   The AFB was sent for **speciation** and came back
36   positive for **MTB**.

37   On surgical consultation with Drs. Ted Evans and Howard
38   Kaufman, it was felt that a **thoracotomy** should be performed.
39   On March 15 the patient was taken to the operating room
40   for this surgical procedure.

41 Surgery revealed a **necrotic** left upper lobe in the
42 superior segments and many lower segment areas of
43 necrosis and chronic inflammatory changes. The
44 bronchopleural fistula was almost at the **bifurcation** of
45 the main stem left bronchus.

46 The patient underwent a left **pneumonectomy**.

47 Postoperatively, the patient had a slightly complicated
48 course. He had some elevated liver function test
49 results and high spiking fevers. He was given
50 nutrition. A sonogram of his liver did not show any
51 dilated ducts. This condition improved slowly
52 over time.

53 The patient was extubated; and, eventually, he was
54 discharged on April 20 tolerating a regular diet and
55 taking antituberculous medications as an outpatient.

56 The patient is to follow up in surgery and medical clinic.

57 _____
58 Valerie Elliott, MD

59 VE/urs

60 d: 4/20/—
61 t: 4/20/—   Word Count 442
62 📼   DSRESSS.1

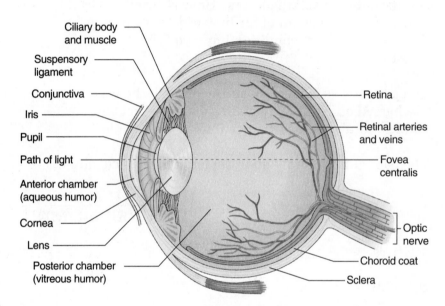

Ciliary body and muscle

Suspensory ligament

Conjunctiva

Iris

Pupil

Path of light

Anterior chamber (aqueous humor)

Cornea

Lens

Posterior chamber (vitreous humor)

Retina

Retinal arteries and veins

Fovea centralis

Optic nerve

Choroid coat

Sclera

Lateral view of eyeball interior

palp	Palpation; indirect measurement of blood pressure (diastolic blood pressure cannot be determined by this method).
bone abscess	Suppuration (pus formation) of articular end of a bone.
saphenous vein	Pertaining to or associated with a saphenous vein in the leg.
Foley	Urinary catheter.
C	Cervical (spine).
AP	Anteroposterior.
intracranial hemorrhage	The escape of blood from a ruptured vessel within the cranium.
WBC	White blood cell (count).
H&H	Hemoglobin and hematocrit.
COAG	Coagulation.
SMA-6	Sequential Multiple Analysis—six different serum tests.
abrasion	A wound caused by rubbing or scraping the skin or mucous membranes.
parieto-occipital	Pertaining to the occipital and parietal areas of the skull (back portion of the head).
hyphema	Hemorrhage into the anterior chamber of the eye.
b.i.d.	Twice a day.

1	PATIENT: Susan Ross
2	CHART #:

ADMITTED: 5/25/–

DISCHARGED: 5/28/–

3 HISTORY:
4 This is a 23-year-old female driving in New York City
5 who was involved in a high-speed motor vehicle accident
6 sometime early Monday morning. The patient's car was
7 found off the road with the steering wheel intact, but
8 the windshield was out.

9 Initial blood pressure by EMS was 100/**palp**. The
10 patient was transported to the emergency room where a
11 large **bone abscess** was obtained and cut down on the
12 right **saphenous vein**.

13 It was noted that the patient had a right dilated fixed
14 pupil. A **Foley** was placed, and x-rays taken of the
15 chest, lateral **C** spine, pelvis, **AP**, and skull.
16 The x-rays were negative.

17 The patient was transported for a CAT scan of the head
18 and abdomen. The CAT scan showed no **intracranial**
19 **hemorrhage** or mass effect of the head, and the abdomen
20 and pelvis were negative for any blood or injury.

21 PAST MEDICAL HISTORY:
22 Negative.

23 LABORATORY EXAMINATION:
24 **WBC** 9.9, **H&H** 13/40, **COAG** normal, **SMA-6** normal.

25 PHYSICAL EXAMINATION:
26 There was a large **abrasion** over the right eye, and
27 large abrasions over the **parieto-occipital** area.
28 The patient's respirations were spontaneous.
29 Her abdomen was soft, and rectal exam showed no
30 heme-positive stool.

31 The extremities had multiple superficial abrasions.

32 HOSPITAL COURSE:
33 The patient was evaluated by ophthalmology who felt
34 that she had **hyphema** of the right eye and Tobrex drops
35 were prescribed.

PATIENT: Susan Ross
CHART #:
Page 2

36 The patient was admitted to the surgical intensive care
37 unit for observation of her neurological status and her
38 right eye.

39 Her laboratory exams all remained within normal limits,
40 and her vital signs were stable.

41 Ophthalmology re-evaluated the eye and felt that it had
42 improved over a 24-hour period. She was transferred to
43 the 4th floor. Plastic surgery also continued its
44 evaluation following plastic surgery of the facial
45 lacerations. Bacitracin was recommended for the sewn
46 lacerations. The patient also received a facial series
47 which were all negative for fractures.

48 Re-evaluation by ophthalmology indicated that the
49 hyphema of the right eye was much improved. The
50 patient was started on PredForte, one drop to the
51 right eye **b.i.d**.

52 DISPOSITION:
53 On post-trauma day three, the patient was discharged to
54 home with followup with the ophthalmology and plastic
55 surgery clinics.

56 INSTRUCTIONS:
57 Diet: Regular. Activity: Ad lib.
58 Medications: Bacitracin to facial wound, Tobrex to
59 right eye, and PredForte to the right eye.

60
61   _____
                                              Fredrich T. Houser, MD

62 FTH/urs

63 d: 5/28/—
64 t: 5/29/—   Word Count 424
65 🔲   DSSENSR.1

Challenge Reports

Section VIII is the "challenge" section where terminology previews and punctuation cues only are provided learners for 15 medical reports to be transcribed. The reports appear in the Instructor's Manual.

This section contains 15 medical reports with terminology previews and punctuation cues only. The reports include seven body systems and are of various lengths. The instructor will use her or his discretion in assigning the reports to challenge those students who are ready to transcribe them.

The referenced body system, patient's name, code name, word count, and type of report follow:

CHALLENGE REPORTS INDEX

BODY SYSTEM	PATIENT	CODE NAME	WORD COUNT	TYPE OF REPORT
FEM	Veronica Crane	SPFEMVC.1	54	Special Procedure
INT	Karen Fisher	SPINTKF.2	84	Special Procedure
NER	Richard Palmer	SPNERRP.3	97	Special Procedure
MUS	Eric Hoffman	CONMUSEH.1	182	Consultation (Letter)
INT	Christine Mitchell	CONINTCM.2	206	Consultation (Letter)
CAR	Edith Starling	SPCARES.4	208	Special Procedure
INT	Tara Connelly	SPINTTC.7	215	Special Procedure
CAR	Patrick O'Brien	SPCARPO.6	223	Special Procedure
CAR	Eugene Warner	SPCAREW.7	246	Special Procedure
MUS	James Shaughnessy	SPMUSJS.8	247	Special Procedure
FEM	Ranjani Selvadurai	ORFEMRS.1	247	Operative Report
GAS	Theodore Lieberman	SPGASTL.9	251	Special Procedure
NER	Ann Newton	CONNERAN.3	263	Consultation (Letter)
GEN	Charlene Tully	SPGENCT.10	296	Special Procedure
MUS	Arthur Sanchez	HPEMUSAS.1	333	History and Physical Examination

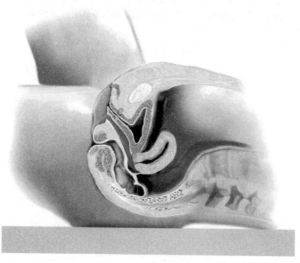

Normal

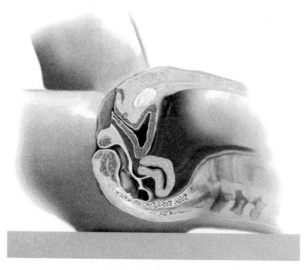

Retroflexed

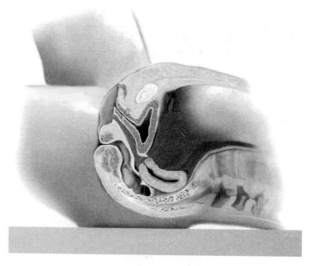

Retroverted

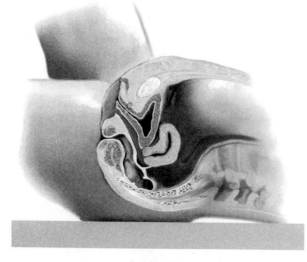

Anteflexed

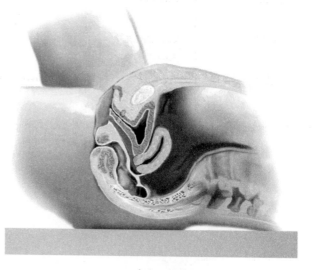

Anteverted

Malposition of uterus

retroverted uterus		Displacement of uterus backward with the cervix pointing forward toward the symphysis pubis.
peritoneal		Concerning the peritoneum (the serous membrane reflected over the viscera and lining the abdominal cavity).
dilatation		Expansion of an organ or vessel.
bilateral		Affecting/relating to two sides.
patent		Wide open; evident; accessible.

NO PUNCTUATION REFERENCES

SPINTKF.1	Karen Fisher	Terminology Preview
turbid		Cloudy; not clear.
aspirated		Drawn in or out by suction.
cytology		The science that deals with the formation, structure, and function of cells.

PUNCTUATION REFERENCES

Line 2	comma—Rule 7
Line 2	hyphen—Rule 1
Line 4	comma—Rule 2
Line 6	hyphen—Rule 4

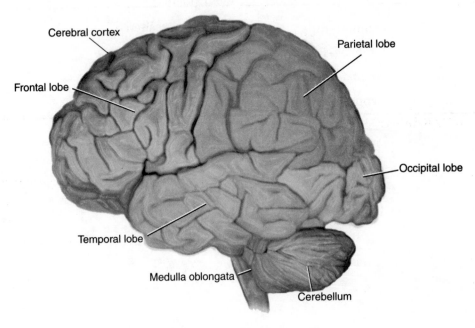

Cerebral cortex

Frontal lobe

Parietal lobe

Occipital lobe

Temporal lobe

Medulla oblongata

Cerebellum

Lateral view of external brain structure

portably		Refers to transportability.
electrode		In electrotherapy an electrode is an instrument with a point or a surface from which to discharge current to the body of the patient.
frontotemporal		Pertaining to the frontal and temporal bones (forehead).
EEG		Electroencephalogram.
bihemispheric		Pertaining to both sides of the cerebral hemisphere.
diffuse		Spreading, scattered.

PUNCTUATION REFERENCE

Line 9	comma—Rule 10

transaxial	Across the long axis of a structure or part.
coronal	Pertaining to front and back images.
sagittal	Pertaining to right and left halves of the body.
talus	The ankle bone articulating with the tibia, fibula, calcaneus, and navicular bone.
delineated	Outlined.
articular	Pertaining to the joints.
effusion	Escape of fluid into a part.
mortise	Ankle joint.
malleoli (pl.) malleolus (s.)	The protuberance on both sides of the ankle joint, the lower extremity of the fibula being known as the lateral malleolus and lower end of the tibia as the medial malleolus.
calcaneus	The heel bone.
Achilles tendon	The tendon of the gastrocnemius and soleus muscles of the leg.
trochlea	The articular smooth surface of a bone upon which glides another bone.
osteochondritis	Inflammation of bone and cartilage.
necrosis	Death of areas of tissue or bone surrounded by healthy parts.

PUNCTUATION REFERENCE

| Line 17 | two commas—Rule 1 |

| --- | --- | --- |
parenchymal		Pertaining to the parenchyma (the essential parts of an organ that are concerned with its function in contradistinction to its framework).
MLO		Medial lateral oblique.
focal		Pertaining to a focus (the point of convergence of light rays or waves of sound).
inferior		Lower.

PUNCTUATION REFERENCES

Line 11	comma—Rule 3
Line 14	hyphen—Rule 1
Line 17	comma—Rule 7
Line 18	comma—Rule 2
Line 18	hyphen—Rule 1

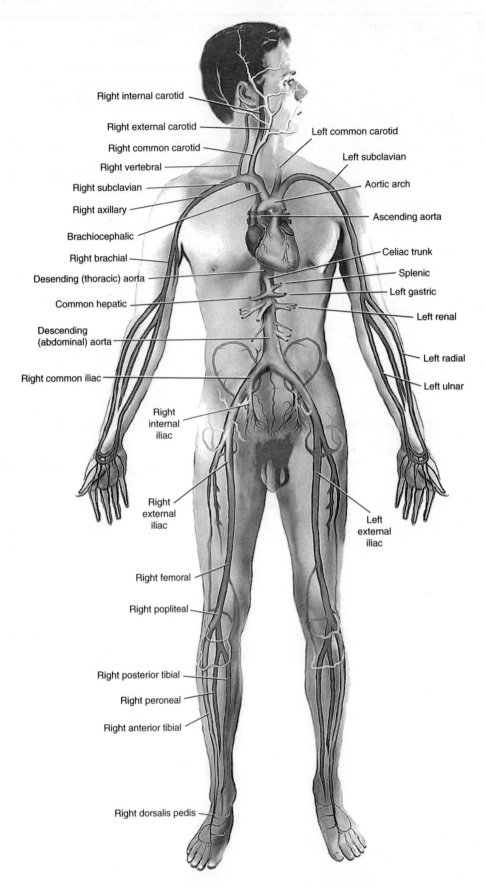

Right internal carotid

Right external carotid

Right common carotid

Right vertebral

Right subclavian

Right axillary

Brachiocephalic

Right brachial

Desending (thoracic) aorta

Common hepatic

Descending (abdominal) aorta

Right common iliac

Right internal iliac

Right external iliac

Right femoral

Right popliteal

Right posterior tibial

Right peroneal

Right anterior tibial

Right dorsalis pedis

Left common carotid

Left subclavian

Aortic arch

Ascending aorta

Celiac trunk

Splenic

Left gastric

Left renal

Left radial

Left ulnar

Left external iliac

Major arteries of the systemic circulation

femoral		Pertaining to the thigh bone, or femur.
ascending		Upward.
oblique		Slanting, diagonal.
carotid		Pertaining to the right and left common carotid arteries, both of which arise from the aorta and are the principal means of blood supply to the head and neck.
vertebral		Pertaining to the vertebral column.
elongated		Extended, lengthened.
stenosis		Constriction or narrowing of a passage or orifice.
bifurcation		A separation into two branches; the point of forking.
atherosclerotic		A form of arteriosclerosis characterized by a variable combination of changes of the intima (the innermost wall of an artery) of arteries (including formation of plaque).
plaque		Formation of deposits of fats in lining of an artery.

PUNCTUATION REFERENCES

Line 2	hyphen—Rule 1
Line 8	comma—Rule 7
Line 11	comma—Rule 7

oblique	Slanting, diagonal
craniocaudal	Direction from head to foot.
microcalcification	One-millionth of a unit (organic tissue that has become hardened by deposition of lime salts in the tissues).
fibroadenomas	Fatty tumors with fibrous tissue forming dense stroma (foundation-supporting tissues of an organ—opposite of parenchyma).
intramammary	Within the breast.
palpable	Perceptible by touch.

PUNCTUATION REFERENCES

Line 10	hyphen—Rule 1
Line 12	comma—Rule 10

SPCARPO.2	Patrick O'Brien	Terminology Preview
sequential		Characterized by regular succession of one thing after another.
occlusion		Closure or state of being closed of a passage.
iliac		Pertaining to the ilium (one of the bones of each half of the pelvis).
hypogastric		Pertaining to the lower middle of the abdomen or hypogastrium.
popliteal		Concerning the posterior surface of the knee.
trifurcation		Division into three branches.

PUNCTUATION REFERENCES

Line 2	hyphen—Rule 1
Line 4	comma—Rule 7
Line 6	comma—Rule 7
Line 10	comma—Rule 7

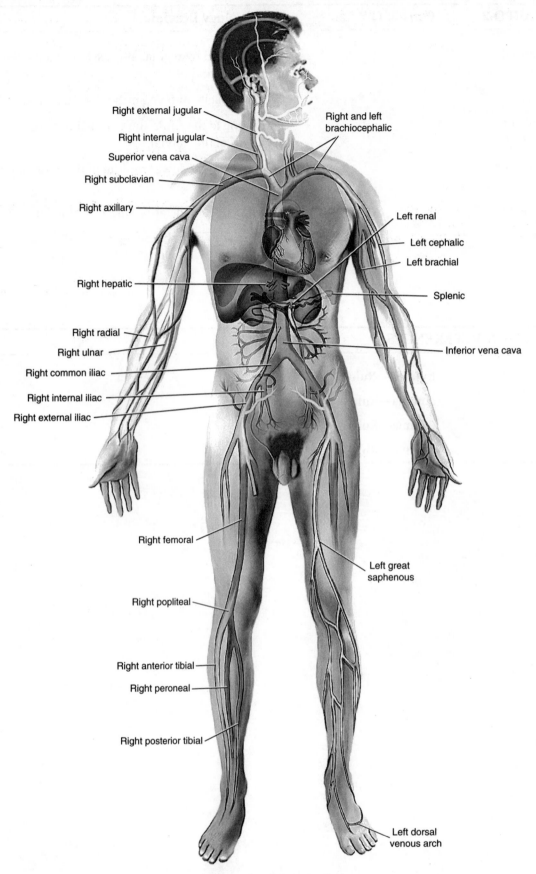

Right external jugular

Right internal jugular

Superior vena cava

Right subclavian

Right axillary

Right hepatic

Right radial

Right ulnar

Right common iliac

Right internal iliac

Right external iliac

Right and left brachiocephalic

Left renal

Left cephalic

Left brachial

Splenic

Inferior vena cava

Right femoral

Left great saphenous

Right popliteal

Right anterior tibial

Right peroneal

Right posterior tibial

Left dorsal venous arch

Major veins of the body

venogram	A roentgenogram (radiographic picture) of the veins.
renal	Pertaining to the kidney.
Omnipaque	Nonionic contrast medium.

PUNCTUATION REFERENCES

| Line 2 | comma—Rule 7 |
| Line 16 | comma—Rule 10 |

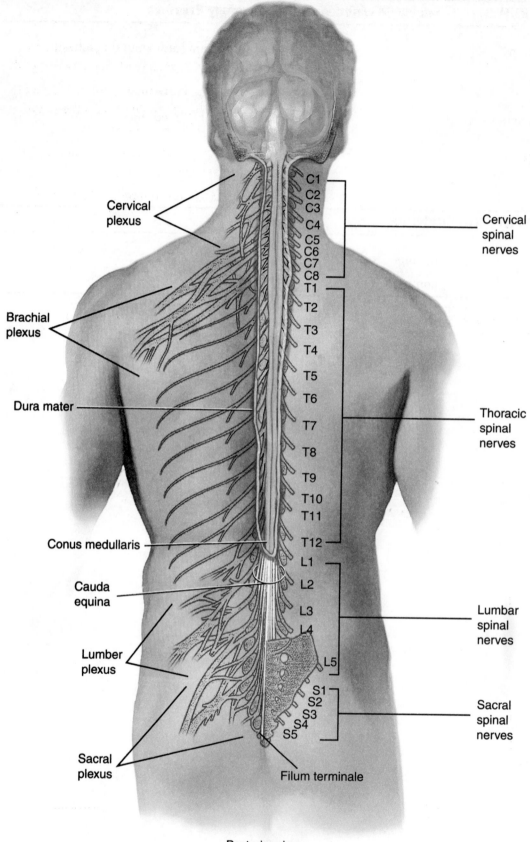

Cervical plexus

Brachial plexus

Dura mater

Conus medullaris

Cauda equina

Lumber plexus

Sacral plexus

C1
C2
C3
C4
C5
C6
C7
C8

Cervical spinal nerves

T1
T2
T3
T4
T5
T6
T7
T8
T9
T10
T11
T12

Thoracic spinal nerves

L1
L2
L3
L4
L5

Lumbar spinal nerves

S1
S2
S3
S4
S5

Sacral spinal nerves

Filum terminale

Posterior view

Posterior view of spinal cord

thecal	Pertaining to a sheath (a covering structure of connective tissue, usually of an elongated part).
thoracolumbar	Pertaining to the thoracic and lumbar parts of the spine, noting their ganglia and the fibers of the sympathetic nervous system.
osteophyte	A bony excrescence (outgrowth), usually branched in shape.
focal	Pertaining to the starting point of a disease process.

PUNCTUATION REFERENCES

Line 2	hyphen—Rule 4
Line 4	hyphen—Rule 1

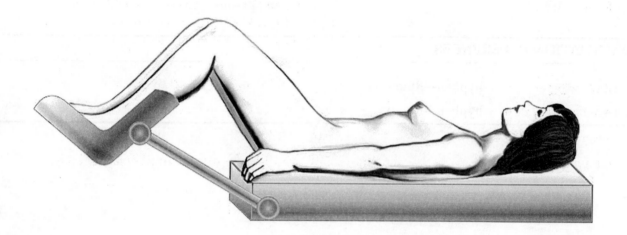

Lithotomy position

verrucous	Wartlike, with raised portions.
carcinoma	Malignant tumor.
endotracheal	Within the trachea.
ovoid	Egg-shaped.
brachytherapy	In radiation therapy, the use of implants of radioactive materials such as radium, cesium, iridium, or gold at the site.
lithotomy	Position in which the patient lies upon the back with thighs flexed upon abdomen and legs upon thighs, which are abducted.
fornix (uteri)	Anterior and posterior spaces into which the upper vagina is divided. These recesses are formed by protrusion of the cervix uteri into the vagina.
paravaginal	Located close to or around the vagina.
adnexa	Ovaries and fallopian tubes.
sutured	Stitched surgically.
circumferentially	Pertaining to the perimeter of an object or body.

PUNCTUATION REFERENCES

Line 10	comma—Rule 7
Line 11	comma—Rule 7
Line 15	comma—Rule 3
Line 17	comma—Rule 7
Line 18	two hyphens—Rule 1
Line 19	comma—Rule 3

midaxillary	Pertaining to the midaxis of the body (a real or imaginary line that runs through the center of a body or about which a part revolves).
subcostal	Below the ribs.
opacification	Shadiness (dense—not transparent).
intrahepatic	Within the liver.
stricture	A narrowing or constriction.
tortuosity	Twisted.
lumen	The space within a tube (or an artery, vein, intestine).
neoplasm	A tumor or growth.
residual	Pertaining to a remainder of something (in this case, the contrast fluid).
Endoscopic Retrograde Cholangiopancreatogram	Radiographic imaging of the bile ducts and pancreas using an endoscope with contrast medium.
costochondral	Pertaining to a rib and its cartilage.

PUNCTUATION REFERENCES

Line 2	hyphen—Rule 1
Line 3	hyphen—Rule 4
Line 8	comma—Rule 7

transaxial	Across the long axis of a structure or part.
subcortical	Below the cortex (outer layer of organ as distinguished from the inner medulla).
periventricular	Around one of the brain's ventricles (cavities).
cerebellar peduncle	A band of fibers connecting parts of the brain.
heterogeneity	Being of unlike nature/quality.
ganglia	Plural of ganglion (a mass of nervous tissue composed principally of nerve-cell bodies and lying outside the brain or spinal cord).
gadolinium	A chemical element of the lathanide group.
Magnevist	Radiopaque agent.
infarct	An area of tissue in an organ or part that undergoes necrosis (death of areas of tissue surrounded by healthy parts) following cessation of blood supply.

PUNCTUATION REFERENCES

Line 10	one comma—Rule 2
Line 10	hyphen—Rule 4
Line 16	comma—Rule 2
Line 18	comma—Rule 7
Line 19	hyphen—Rule 4

calyceal		Pertaining to the calyces (plural of calyx, a cuplike organ or cavity).
pyelogram		A roentgenogram of the ureter and renal pelvis.
percutaneous		Effected through the skin.
nephrostomy		Formation of an artificial fistula into the renal pelvis.
extravasation		Escape of fluids into surrounding tissue.
perinephric		Around the kidney.
ureteropelvic		Pertaining to the ureter and pelvis.

PUNCTUATION REFERENCES

Line 4	comma—Rule 3
Line 6	semicolon—Rule 10
Line 7	comma—Rule 3
Line 9	comma—Rule 3
Line 11	comma—Rule 3
Line 12	comma—Rule 3
Line 14	two commas—Rule 10
Line 15	semicolon—Rule 1

atrial fibrillation	Extremely rapid, incomplete contractions of the atria resulting in fine, rapid, irregular, and uncoordinated movements.
hyperlipidemia	Excessive quantity of fat in the blood.
palpitation	Rapid, violent, or throbbing pulsation, as an abnormally rapid throbbing or fluttering of the heart.
dyspnea	Labored or difficult breathing, sometimes accompanied by pain.
syncope	A transient loss of consciousness due to inadequate blood flow to the brain.
dementia	A broad (global) impairment of intellectual function (cognition) that usually is progressive and that interferes with normal social and occupational activities.
bruits	An adventitious sound of venous or arterial origin heard on auscultation.
percussion	Use of the fingertips to tap the body lightly but sharply to determine position, size, and consistency of an underlying structure and the presence of fluid or pus in a cavity.
auscultation	Process of listening for sounds within the body, usually those of thoracic or abdominal viscera, in order to detect some abnormal condition.
myocardial ischemia	Insufficient blood supply to the heart.
hypercholesterolemia	Excessive amount of cholesterol in the blood.
telemetry	Transmission of data electronically to a distant location.
Cardizem	Calcium channel blocking agent.
titrated	Estimated by titration (estimation of the concentration of a chemical solution by adding known amounts of standard reagents until alteration in color or electrical state occurs).
digoxin	A heart stimulant.
atenolol	Beta-adrenergic blocking agent.
ischemia	Local and temporary deficiency of blood supply due to obstruction of the circulation to a part.
prophylaxis	Observance of rules necessary to prevent disease.
anticoagulated	Blood coagulation delayed or prevented.

PUNCTUATION REFERENCES

Line 4	two hyphens—Rule 1
Line 8	two commas—Rule 1
Line 12	three commas—Rule 1
Line 12	apostrophe—Rule 1
Line 16	three commas—Rule 1
Line 24	three commas—Rule 1
Line 30	comma—Rule 3
Line 34	comma—Rule 3
Line 35	semicolon—Rule 1

APPENDIXES

Learning About Medical Terminology

Your goal as you learn terminology is to analyze the word parts, which will make the understanding of complex terminology easier. You divide words into basic units containing roots, prefixes, suffixes, and combining vowels.

When you break down medical terms into their respective parts, start with the suffix, then go to the root, and follow through with the prefix, if applicable.

EXAMPLE: cardiology cardi/o/logy
The suffix **-logy** means **process of study.**
The root **cardi** means **heart.**
The combining vowel **o** links **root to suffix.**
Definition: The process of the study of the heart.

EXAMPLE: cardiomegaly cardi/o/megaly
The suffix **-megaly** means **enlargement.**
The root **cardi** means **heart.**
The combining vowel **o** links **root to suffix.**
Definition: The enlargement of the heart.

EXAMPLE: electrocardiogram electr/o/cardi/o/gram
The suffix **-gram** means **record.**
The root **electr** means **electricity.**
The root **cardi** means **heart.**
The combining vowel **o** links **root to root to suffix.**
Definition: The record of the electricity of the heart.

EXAMPLE: gastroenterology gastr/o/enter/o/logy
The suffix **-logy** means **process of study.**
The root **gastr** means **stomach.**
The root **enter** means **intestines.**
The combining vowel **o** links **root to root to suffix.**
Definition: The process of the study of the stomach and intestines.

EXAMPLE: epigastric epi/gastr/ic
The suffix **-ic** means **pertaining to.**
The prefix **epi-** means **above.**
The root **gastr** means **stomach.**
Definition: Pertaining to above the stomach.

EXAMPLE: hepatitis hepat/itis
The suffix **-itis** means **inflammation.**
The root **hepat** means **liver.**
Definition: Inflammation of the liver.

EXAMPLE: sacral sacr/al
The suffix **-al** means **pertaining to.**
The root **sacr** means **sacrum.**
Definition: Pertaining to the sacrum (lower back).

EXAMPLE: arthralgia arthr/algia
The suffix **-algia** means **pain.**
The root **arthr** means **joint.**
Definition: Pain in the joint.

EXAMPLE: bradycardia brady/card/ia
The suffix **-ia** means **condition.**
The prefix **brady-** means **slow.**
The root **card** means **heart.**
Definition: Condition of slow heart (beat).

Prefixes, Suffixes, Roots

A prefix is a word part found at the beginning of a word; it is never used alone. Awareness of what a prefix means often leads to understanding of the full word. For example, postoperative = post (after), or after an operation.

Prefixes Commonly Used in Medical Terms

Prefix	Meaning
a, an	no; not; without
ab	away from
ad	toward
ana	up; apart; excessive
ante	before; forward
anti	against
auto	self
bi	two
brachy	short
brady	slow
cata	down
con	together; with
contra	against; opposite
de	lack of; down
dia	complete; through
dys	bad; painful; difficult
ec	out; outside
ecto	out; outside
em	in
en	in; within
endo	in; within
epi	above; upon; on
eso	inward
eu	good
ex	out; away from
poly	many
post	after; behind
pre	before; in front of

Prefix	Meaning
pro	before
re	back
retro	behind
semi	half
sub	under; below
supra	above
sym	together; with
syn	together; with
tachy	fast
tetra	four
trans	across
tri	three
ultra	beyond; excess
uni	one

A suffix is a word part found at the end of a word. Knowledge of the meaning of a suffix can often help the transcriptionist figure out the meaning of the entire word. For example, tonsillitis = tonsil + itis (inflammation), or an inflammation of the tonsils.

Suffixes Commonly Used in Medical Terms

Suffix	Meaning
ac	pertaining to
agia	excessive pain
al	pertaining to
algia	pain
ar	pertaining to
ary	pertaining to
cele	hernia
crine	secrete; separate
crit	separate
cyesis	pregnancy
cyte	cell
dynia	pain
eal	pertaining to
ectomy	removal; excision
emia	blood
er	one who
fusion	to pour
grade	to go
gram	record
graph	instrument for recording
ia	condition
iac	pertaining to
ic	pertaining to

Suffix	Meaning
ism	process
ist	specialist
itis	inflammation
logy	study of
megaly	enlargement
meter	measure
oid	resembling
ole	little; small
oma	tumor; mass
opsy	view of
or	one who
osis	abnormal condition
ous	pertaining to
pathy	disease
penia	deficiency
pexy	fixation; to put in place
phagia	eating; swallowing
plasty	surgical repair
pnea	breathing
ptosis	drooping; sagging; prolapse
rrhage	bursting forth of blood
rrhea	flow; discharge
scope	instrument for visual examination
sis	state of; condition
spasm	sudden contraction of muscles
stomy	new opening
therapy	treatment
thorax	pleural cavity; chest
tic	pertaining to
tome	instrument to cut
tomy	process of cutting
ule	little; small
uria	urination; urine
us	thing
y	condition; process

Roots Commonly Used in Medical Terms

A word root is the foundation of the word. The medical language is logical, and each term can be broken down into its basic component parts and then understood. For example, gastralgia (algia/pain) and gastr (root for stomach) = stomach pain or stomach ache. Combining vowels are usually retained between two roots in a word even if the second root begins with a vowel. For example, gastroenteric (gastr-root-stomach), (enter-root-intestines), (ic-suffix-pertaining to) + combining vowel o = gastroenteric (pertaining to the stomach and intestines).

Root/Combining Form	Meaning
abdomin/o	abdomen
aden/o	gland
adren/o	adrenal glands
alveol/o	alveolus; air sac; small sac
amni/o	amnion
angi/o	vessel
arteri/o	artery
arthr/o	joint
audi/o	hearing
axill/o	armpit
brachi/o	arm
bronch/o	bronchial tube
carcin/o	cancerous
cardi/o	heart
caud/o	tail; lower part of body
cauter/o	heat; burn
cephal/o	head
chol/e	bile; gall
clavicul/o	clavicle (collar bone)
crani/o	skull
crin/o	secrete
cyan/o	blue
derm/o	skin
dips/o	thirst
dors/o	back (of body)
ech/o	sound
enter/o	intestines
eti/o	cause
femor/o	femur (thigh bone)
furc/o	forking; branching
gastro/o	stomach
gloss/o	tongue
gravid/o	pregnancy
gynec/o	woman; female
hepat/o	liver
hydr/o	water

Root/Combining Form	Meaning
inguin/o	groin
lact/o	milk
laryng/o	larynx (voice box)
mamm/o	breast
medi/o	middle
metacarp/o	metacarpals (hand bones)
necr/o	death
nephr/o	kidney
onc/o	tumor
ophthlm/o	eye
orth/o	straight
ov/o	egg
ovari/o	ovary
path/o	disease
pector/o	chest
phag/o	eat; swallow
pharyng/o	throat; pharynx
rect/o	rectum
rhin/o	nose
secti/o	to cut
splen/o	spleen
stomat/o	mouth
thorac/o	chest
tonsil/o	tonsil
ur/o	urine; urinary tract
uter/o	uterus; womb
ventr/o	belly side of body
vertebr/o	vertebrae (backbone)
vesic/o	urinary bladder
xiph/o	sword

PUNCTUATION REFERENCES

Possessive Case (Use of the Apostrophe)

The Comma

The Dash

The Hyphen

The Semicolon

Quotation Marks

Capitalization Rules

POSSESSIVE CASE

Possessive case indicates possession or ownership. Possessive nouns express something that is part of a person, place, thing, or idea. For example, *patient's medication* shows that the patient is the owner of the medication. *Medication* is the noun that follows the possessive noun, *patient's*. To check the accuracy of the possessive, change the words to *the medication of the patient*.

Use an apostrophe (') to form the possessive. The rules for forming a possessive noun are as follows:

---

1. To form the possessive of singular nouns, add an apostrophe *s* ('s) to the noun. The word that has the apostrophe is the word that owns something.

   patient's bed [the bed of the patient]
   doctor's white coat [the white coat of the doctor]

2. The possessive of plural nouns ending in s is formed by adding only an apostrophe after the *s* (s').

   doctors' dressing room [the dressing rooms of the doctors]
   nurses' scrub gowns [the scrub gowns of the nurses]

   If the plural word does not end in *s*, add an apostrophe and the letter *s* ('s).

   children's diseases [the diseases of children]

3. Irregular nouns not ending in s need an apostrophe *s* ('s) to form the possessive.

   The *children's* ward is on the fourth floor.
   The *women's* lounge is down the hall.

4. If two people own an item, only the last name takes the possessive form.

   Lorry and Doreen's book on *Grammar and Writing Skills for the Health Professional* is on the shelf.

   If each person owns the item, both names take the possessive form.

   Dr. Archie's and *Dr. Villes's* stethoscopes are on the treatment table.

5. To form the possessive of singular nouns ending in *s,* add an apostrophe and an *s* ('s).

   Mr. Jones's daughter.

6. To form the possessive of plural nouns ending in *s,* only add an apostrophe (').

   The *Jones'* families.

THE COMMA

Within sentences, the comma is the most frequently used punctuation mark. It is also the punctuation mark that causes the most difficulty. Errors fall into two extreme categories: Commas are either disregarded or they are used too frequently. The main purpose of the comma is to group words that belong together and separate words that do not. A comma also represents a brief pause when reading. The best rule is to follow about commas is not to use it unless there is a reason to do so.

Rule 1: The comma is used to separate three or more items in a series.

Examples

Coryza, cough, and sore throat are common in the winter.

Influenza is characterized by the sudden onset of *chills, headache, and myalgia.*

The five stages of grieving are *denial, anger, bargaining, depression, and acceptance.*

If items in a series are each linked by *and* or *or*, a comma is not used.

Examples

The four blood types are A *and* B *and* AB *and* O.

You could give 10 mg *or* 20 mg *or* 40 mg of Demerol I.M. for the pain.

Rule 2: Use a comma to separate two or more adjectives that describe the same noun.

Examples

Purulent, rusty-colored sputum was taken to the lab for testing.

The x-ray revealed *numerous, questionable nodules.*

Rule 3: A comma is used between two independent clauses joined by coordinating conjunctions (*and, but, or, not, for, so, yet*).

Examples

Medicare is administered by the Social Security Administration, *but the public welfare office handles Medicaid.*

Patients usually recover rapidly from influenza, *yet some patients experience lassitude for weeks.*

Did you hear about the new medication for arthritis, *and how it affects the elderly?*

Rule 4: Place a comma between the day and year. If a date is used in a sentence, a comma goes between the year and the rest of the sentence.

Examples

February 28, 2009

On *February 28, 2009*, the hospital will review its policies.

Rule 5: Use a comma between the city and state. When the city and state are used in a sentence, a comma is placed after the state.

Examples

Boston, Massachusetts

Anesthesia was first discovered in *Boston, Massachusetts*, at Massachusetts General Hospital.

The American Association of Medical Assistants and the American Medical Associations are located in *Chicago, IL.*

Rule 6: Use a comma to separate numbers that have four or more digits.

3,000 30,000 300,000 3,000,000

Exceptions include addresses and year numbers of four digits.

The address is *3600* Main Street.

Rule 7: Use a comma to separate appositives, nouns of direct address, titles that follow a person's name, and introductory words from the rest of the sentence.

Examples

Doctor, please listen carefully to what I have to say.

Please listen carefully, *Doctor*, to what I have to say.

Yes, you may have a regular diet.

However, I do think you will have to curtail your intake of cholesterol.

A decrease in total dietary fat will help, *however*.

Dr. Villes, *a pathologist*, graduated from a medical school in Burlington, VT.

The pathologist, *Norm Villes, M.D.*, graduated from a medical school in Burlington, VT.

Rule 8: Use a comma to separate clauses and phrases that are unnecessary to the meaning of a sentence (nonessential, or nonrestrictive, clauses and phrases).

Examples

The hospital, *unlike most facilities*, has a comprehensive evacuation plan.
[*Unlike most facilities* is not necessary to the meaning of the sentence.]

The hourly pay, *in some circumstances*, increases over a period of time.
[The sentence still makes sense when *in some circumstances* is omitted.]

Programs, *which are available on request*, are free of charge.

The healing was satisfactory, *treated with antibiotics*.

Rule 9: A comma follows the salutation in a friendly letter and the complimentary close.

Examples

Yours truly,   *Sincerely,*   *Best regards,*

Dear friend,   *Hello, Bill,*

Rule 10: Separate parenthetical expressions with a comma, depending on where they are placed in the sentence. Parenthetical expressions include

I believe (*think, hope, see,* etc.)		*I am sure*	*on the contrary*
on the other hand	*after all*	*by the way*	*incidentally*
in fact	*indeed*	*naturally*	*of course*
in my opinion	*for example*	*however*	*nonetheless*
to tell the truth			

Examples

The surgery was successful. *Therefore,* there is no need of further treatment.

The report, *I hope,* will give you many options about treatments.

In my opinion, the signs and symptoms are indicative of angina pectoris.

An inadequate supply of oxygen to the myocardium, *for example,* is caused by arteriosclerosis.

Rule 11: Use a comma to separate a direct quotation.

Examples

The doctor said, "*You must give up smoking.*"

"I really don't have the courage," the patient replied.

"In that case," the doctor continued, *"you sign your own death warrant."*

Rule 12: A comma is used to set off contrasting statements that are introduced by the words *not, rather,* and *though.*

Examples

Right now, *rather* than later, increase the medication.

I would describe her mood as thoughtful, *not* sullen.

THE DASH

The purpose of the dash (—) is to set off unnecessary items from the rest of the sentence. The reason for using the dash, rather than any other punctuation mark, is to give more emphasis to words. The dash may be applied singly or in pairs. However, it is rarely seen in medical documentation.

Examples

I have 30 years—*very rewarding ones*—of medical practice.

The forms are to be written exclusively by physicians—*not nurses, not therapists, not social workers, and not aides.*

THE HYPHEN

The following rules cover the use of hyphens; however, some hyphenated terms become one word over time. Be sure to consult a dictionary when in doubt about hyphens.

Rule 1: Use a hyphen between compound words used as an adjective when the adjective precedes the noun.

Examples

all-day surgery	*102-year-old* man	*grayish-black* tissue
follow-up	*one-by-one*	

A *well-developed, well-nourished* young man.

A *34-year-old* male was admitted to the West Wing.

When a compound word follows a noun, it is not hyphenated.

The young man was *well developed.*

Compound words that have become commonly used are not hyphenated.

earache   *gallbladder*   *nosebleed*

Rule 2: Use a hyphen with numbers 21 to 99 and with written fractions.

thirty-five days ago   *one-third of the hospital rooms*

Rule 3: Use a hyphen with a prefix added to a word that begins with a capital letter.

mid-March   *un-American*

Rule 4: Some adjective forms are always hyphenated, whether before or after the nouns they modify.

self-conscious   *cross-referenced*

Rule 5: Use a hyphen in some compound words used as nouns.

mother-in-law   *ex-employer*

Always consult the dictionary when in doubt about hyphenation.

THE SEMICOLON

The seimcolon is a punctuation mark that is stronger than a comma; that is, it indicates a more definite break in the flow of a sentence. Semicolons join items that are grammatically alike or closely related.

Rule 1: A semicolon is used instead of a comma and a coordinating conjunction (*and, but, or, nor, for, yet* and *so*) to separate two independent clauses.

Examples

A physician shall respect the law; recognize the responsibility to change any law that is contrary to the best interest of the patient.

Almost all victims of violence go to emergency centers; many have no health insurance.

Many people are homeless because they were discharged from a mental institution; most are without proper follow-up health care.

If a coordinating conjunction is present, commas are used to separate independent clauses. The clauses can also be rewritten as two sentences.

Examples

The cost of health care in the U.S. is out of control; 37 million have no health insurance and 35 million are underinsured.

The cost of health care in the U.S. is out of control, yet 37 million have no health insurance and 35 million are underinsured.

The cost health care in the U.S. is out of control. Thirty-seven million have no health insurance and thirty-five million are underinsured.

Rule 2: Use a semicolon between independent clauses when the second clause begins with a transitional expression such as:

for example	*for instance*	*otherwise*
that is	*besides*	*therefore*
accordingly	*moreover*	*consequently*
nevertheless	*furthermore*	*however*
instead	*hence*	*namely*

Examples

Every medical office has its unique pathology format; *however,* the data required is the same.

The arterial blood gas reports are good; *therefore,* we can begin the process of weaning from the ventilator.

The cardiac rate was rapid and regular; *consequently,* there are no extrasystoles.

The patient was afebrile after admission; *nevertheless,* he became febrile with recurrent episodes of pain in the left side of the chest.

Note: A comma sets off one independent clause: "*The medical report is completed,* all ten pages." A semicolon sets off two independent clauses: "The medical report is completed; mail it first class."

Rule 3: Use a semicolon with a series of items that have one or more commas.

Examples

Those present at the meeting were Dr. M. P. Carr, my family physician; Mrs. P. Archy, my lawyer; Bob, my husband; and Valerie, my daughter.

I sent copies to Burlington, Vermont; Concord, New Hampshire; and Boston, Massachusetts.

QUOTATION MARKS

Quotation marks are used to enclose the exact words of the speaker. Quotations are often used in the subjective part of a problem-oriented medical record (POMR) charting, or when it is necessary to quote the exact words of the patient or a family member.

Examples

Robert said, *"I have pain in my chest."* [The period goes inside the quotation mark when words apply only to the quoted material.]

"I go to physical therapy at 3 p.m.," said Sheila. [Note the comma *inside* the quote.]

"Take the patient to room 205," Robert said, *"while I bring the chart to the desk."* [Note the interruption of the quotation.]

"What was the fasting blood sugar?" asked Dr. Oberg. [Note the question mark *inside* the quote.]

"I would advise caution," said the physician, *"because your condition is serious."*

Quotation marks are also used to enclose a part of a completed published work or to indicate that words or phrases are being used in a special way.

Examples

Chapter 9 is titled "Punctuation."

The title of the seminar is "Stress Management."

Write "confidential" on the envelope.

CAPITALIZATION RULES

Capitalize the following except as noted:

The pronoun *I*	After *I* read the book, you can have it.
The first word in a sentence	*Poems* are made by fools like me.
The first word in any line of poetry	*But* only God can make a tree.
People's names	*Roberta*, *F. Scott Fitzgerald*
Titles as part of a person's name	*Senator* Kennedy, *Prime Minister* Abouti
Do *not* capitalize a title used without a person's name.	secretary of state, the senator from Ohio
Words like mother, father, aunt, uncle used alone.	I asked *Mother* to go.
Do *not* capitalize family members when accompanied by a possessive pronoun.	I asked my *mother* to go.

Title after a name	Jonathan Harlan, *M.D.*, Randy Kane, *Jr.*
Geographic names, streets, towns, and regions of a country.	*C*hina, *D*ade *C*ounty, *W*est *S*ide, the *S*outheast, *R*odeo *D*rive, *F*rance, *A*tlantic *O*cean
Do *not* capitalize directions.	Drive *w*est. Face *s*outh.
Languages, races.	*S*panish, *F*rench accent, *B*lack history
Do *not* capitalize *the* before these names.	*t*he Nile River, *t*he French people
Important buildings or structures	Vietnam *M*emorial, *T*rump *T*ower
Historical ages, events	*R*omantic *E*ra, *S*enior *P*rom
Do *not* capitalize *the* before these names.	*t*he Senior Prom
Names of products	*A*von, *B*ayer
Names of companies, stores banks	*D*elta *A*irlines, *M*ercy *M*edical *C*enter, *P*athology *D*epartment, *F*ord truck
Names of specific courses	*E*nglish *G*rammar 101
Do not capitalize subject matter.	*E*nglish grammar
Organizations	*A*merican *M*edical *A*ssociation, *A*merican *A*ssociation for *M*edical *T*ranscription
Political parties	*D*emocrat, *R*epublican
Religions, deity, worshiped figures	*B*aptist, *J*udaism, *C*atholicism, *B*uddha, *C*hrist, *A*llah, *G*od, *B*ible, *P*romised *L*and
Important words in the title of a book, movie, etc.	*B*ill of *R*ights, *G*ray's *A*natomy
Unless they are the first word in a title, a, an, the, of, and, from, to, are not capitalized.	*T*he Grapes *o*f Wrath, *T*he Return *o*f *t*he Native
Holidays, days of the week, months	*C*hristmas, *S*unday, *J*uly, *H*anukkah
Do *not* capitalize seasons.	*s*pring, *s*ummer, *w*inter, *f*all
Do *not* capitalize academic years.	*f*reshman, *s*ophomore, *j*unior, *s*enior
First word in a direct quote	"*T*he pain is here," said Mary. Mary said, "*T*he pain is here."
Do *not* capitalize the first word of the continuation of an interrupted quote.	"The pain," said Mary, "*i*s in the stomach."
Eponyms	*P*arkinson's disease, *B*abinski's reflex, *A*pgar score, *F*owler's position, *B*ell's palsy, *E*pstein-*B*arr virus
Certain acronyms	B.C. Ph.D. A.D.

MEDICAL TRANSCRIPTIONIST SELECTED REFERENCES

ABBREVIATIONS/ACRONYMS

The Charles Press Dictionary of Medical Abbreviations, 6th ed. 2002, Charles Press, Publishers

Dictionary of Medical Acronyms and Abbreviations, 4th ed. (Jablonski), 2001, Hanley & Belfus, Inc.

Medical Abbreviations: 15,000 Conveniences at the Expense of Communications and Safety, 10th ed. (includes free access to Internet version, updated monthly) (Davis), 2001, Neil M. Davis Associates

Melloni's Illustrated Dictionary of Medical Abbreviations (Melloni/Melloni), 1998, Parthenon Publishing Group, Inc.

Stedman's Abbrev: Abbreviations, Acronyms & Symbols, 2nd ed., 1999, Lippincott Williams & Wilkins

Stedman's Abbrev: Abbreviations, Acronyms & Symbols, 2nd ed. (CD-ROM), 2001, Lippincott Williams & Wilkins

ANATOMY/PHYSIOLOGY

Anatomy & Physiology, 6th ed. (Seeley et al.), 2002, McGraw-Hill College Division

Body Structures and Functions, 9th ed. (Scott/Fong), 1998, Delmar Thompson Learning

Delmar's Anatomy & Physiology Challenge CD-ROM (Pucillo), 1998, Delmar Thompson Learning

Fundamentals of Anatomy & Physiology, 5th ed. (Martini), 2001, Prentice-Hall

Hole's Essentials of Human Anatomy & Physiology, 8th ed. (Shier et al.), 2002, McGraw-Hill College Division

The Human Body in Health and Illness, 2nd ed. (Herlihy/Maebius), 2002, W. B. Saunders

Mosby's Handbook of Anatomy and Physiology (Patton/Thibodeau), 2000, Mosby

Stedman's Anatomy & Physiology Words, 2nd ed., 2002, Lippincott Williams & Wilkins

Understanding Human Anatomy & Physiology 4th ed. (Mader), 2001, McGraw-Hill College Division

ELECTRONIC DOCUMENT CREATION

Corel WordPerfect, Corel Corporation, USA

GearXport (for receiving and sending voice and text files), TranscriptionGear.com

MediScribe, 1997 HealthCare Technologies, Inc.

Microsoft Word, Microsoft Corporation

MPWord (word processor designed for medical transcription), Emmaus MedPen

RapidWrite Pro (rapid text entry), Stenograph, L.L.C.

ELECTRONIC HEALTH RECORD STANDARDS

ANNUAL BOOK OF ASTM STANDARDS, Vol. 14.01: Healthcare Informatics Computerized Systems (annual), ASTM

Standard Guide for Confidentiality, Privacy, Access and Data Security Principles for Health Information Including Computer Based Patient Records: E1869–97 (ASTM Subcommittee E31.17), 1997, ASTM

Standard Guide for Content and Structure of the Computer-based Patient Record: E1384–99 (ASTM Subcommittee E31.19), 1999, ASTM

Standard Guide for Management of the Confidentiality and Security of Dictation, Transcription, and Transcribed Health Records: E1902–97 (ASTM Subcommittee E31.22), 1997, ASTM

HEALTH INSURANCE PORTABILITY AND ACCOUNTABILITY ACT (HIPAA)

HIPAA for MTs, version 1.0 Considerations for the Medical Transcriptionist as Business Associate *with* Sample HIPAA Business Associate Agreement, 2002, AAMT

MEDICAL DICTIONARIES

Dorland's Illustrated Medical Dictionary, 29th ed., 2000, W. B. Saunders

Dorland's Electronic Medical Dictionary, 29th ed., 2000, W. B. Saunders

Lexikon: Dictionary of Health Care Terms, Organizations, and Acronyms for the Era of Reform, 2nd ed. (O'Leary et al.), 1997, JCAHO

Merriam-Webster's Medical Audio Dictionary (CD-ROM), 1997, Merriam Webster, Inc.

Merriam-Webster's Medical Desk Dictionary with CD-ROM, 1998, Merriam-Webster, Inc

Mosby's Medical, Nursing, and Allied Health Dictionary, 6th ed., 2002, Mosby

Stedman's Electronic Medical Dictionary, Version 5, 2000, Lippincott Williams & Wilkins

Stedman's Medical Dictionary, 27th ed., 2000, Lippincott Williams & Wilkins

Taber's Cyclopedic Medical Dictionary, 19th ed. (Ed.: Thomas), 2001, F. A. Davis Co.

Taber's Electronic Medical Dictionary, version 2.0, F. A. Davis Co.

Vera Pyle's Current Medical Terminology, 9th ed., 2002, Health Professions Institute

MEDICAL/LEGAL ETHICS

Ethical Dimensions of Health Professions, 3rd ed., (Purtilo), 1999, W. B. Saunders

Legal and Ethical Issues in Health Occupations (Aiken), 2002, W. B. Saunders

Medical Law, Ethics, and Bioethics for Ambulatory Health Care, 4th ed. (Lewis/Tamparo), 1998 F. A. Davis Co.

MEDICAL TRANSCRIPTIONISTS' REFERENCE RESOURCES

Compensation for Medical Transcriptionists, 1999, Hay Group, AAMT

2002 AAMT Desk Companion (published yearly), AAMT

MEDICAL SOFTWARE

Complete Medical/Pharmaceutical Spellchecker, 2002, Sylvan Software

Dorland's Electronic Medical Speller, 29th ed., 2000, W. B. Saunders

MedPen (automation software for MS Word and WordPerfect), 1999, Emmaus MedPen

MP Count (free software for counting and invoicing MS Word documents), 2000, Emmaus MedPen

Stedman's Plus Medical/Pharmaceutical Spellchecker, 2002, Lippincott Williams & Wilkins

Taber's Medical/Pharmaceutical Spell Checker, F. A. Davis Co.

When the Name of the Game is Saving Keystrokes (video and workbook) (Rolland), 1999, Macro-EZ

WP Count, 1997, Productive Performance, Inc.

MEDICAL TERMINOLOGY

Delmar's Comprehensive Medical Terminology (Jones), 1999, Delmar Thompson Learning

Essentials of Medical Terminology, 2nd ed. (Davies), 2002, Delmar Thompson Learning

The Language of Medicine, 6th ed. (Chabner), 2001, W. B. Saunders

Medical Terminology: A Medical Specialty Approach with Patients' Records (Gylys/Wedding), 2002, F. A. Davis Co.

MT Desk (medical word glossary and MT link), www.mtdesk.com

PERIODICALS

ADVANCE for Health Information Professionals (biweekly), Merion Publications, Inc.

HIPAA Compliance Alert (monthly), United Communications Group

In Confidence (monthly), AHIMA

JAAMT (Journal of AAMT) (bimonthly), AAMT

The Latest Word (Ed.: Grow) (bimonthly), W. B. Saunders

MT Monthly (monthly), Computer Systems Management

Perspectives on the Medical Transcription Profession (free magazine) (quarterly), Health Professions Institute

PUNCTUATION AND STYLE GUIDES

The AAMT Book of Style for Medical Transcription, 2nd ed., 2002, AAMT

The Gregg Reference Manual, 9th ed. (Sabin), 2000, McGraw-Hill Glencoe

Medical Transcription Guide: Do's and Don'ts, 2nd ed. (Fordney/Diehl), 1999, W. B. Saunders

The Online English Grammar, www.edunet.com/english/grammar/

Grammar and Writing Skills for the Health Professional, (Villemaire), 2001, Delmar Thompson Learning

SPEECH RECOGNITION

Boomerang, Version 2.0, Dictaphone

MT Meeting Place (speech recognition for MTs), www.mtmeetingplace.com

WEB SITES

AMA Physician Select (online physician finder), www.ama-assn.org/aps/amahg.htm

American Association for Medical Transcription, www.aamt.org

Big Book (includes yellow pages from entire US), www.bigbook.com

MedNexus (web site with medical links), www.mednexus.com/public/mnlinks1.html

Medword (MT links, including transcription services and schools), www.medword.com/mtlist.html

MT Jobs (job searching through MT Daily), www.mtjobs.com

Student Grade Record of Class Transcripts, Quizzes and Transcription Tests

Use the following logs to keep track of your progress

STUDENT GRADE RECORD OF CLASS TRANSCRIPTS, QUIZZES, AND TRANSCRIPTION TESTS

Item Code	Date Submitted	Grade	Date Resubmitted	Grade

STUDENT GRADE RECORD OF CLASS TRANSCRIPTS, QUIZZES, AND TRANSCRIPTION TESTS

Item Code	Date Submitted	Grade	Date Resubmitted	Grade

STUDENT GRADE RECORD OF CLASS TRANSCRIPTS, QUIZZES, AND TRANSCRIPTION TESTS

Item Code	Date Submitted	Grade	Date Resubmitted	Grade

STUDENT GRADE RECORD OF CLASS TRANSCRIPTS, QUIZZES, AND TRANSCRIPTION TESTS

Item Code	Date Submitted	Grade	Date Resubmitted	Grade

STUDENT GRADE RECORD OF CLASS TRANSCRIPTS, QUIZZES, AND TRANSCRIPTION TESTS

Item Code	Date Submitted	Grade	Date Resubmitted	Grade

Index

Note: An "f" following a page number indicates a figure.

D

DC, 342, 343
D&C, 163, 164
Dakin's solution, 301, 302
Dash. *See* Punctuation
Debrided, 326, 327
Debridement, 279, 281, 301, 302, 307, 308
Decadron, 404, 405
Decidual, 199, 200
Decompression, 363, 364
Decubitus, 301, 302
Decubitus ulcer, 307, 308
Defervesced, 391, 393
Defibrillated, 273, 275
Defibrillator, 56, 58
Delineated, 424
Deltoid, 264, 266, 335, 336
Deltopectoral groove, 264, 266
Dementia, 439
Density, 239, 240
Dermis, 268, 269
Descending, 220, 221
Dexamethasone, 39, 41
Dexon, 273, 275, 279, 282
Diabenase, 404, 405
Diabetes mellitus, 163, 164
Diaphragmatic, 366, 368
Diastolic, 197, 198
Diffuse, 231, 232, 423
Digestive system, 91f, 283f
Digital arteries and veins, 323, 324
Digoxin, 439
Dilatation, 47, 50, 236, 237, 374, 375, 420
Dilated, 294, 295, 363, 364
Dilaudid, 353, 354
Discharge summary reports, 339
  cardiovascular, 342–343, 344–346
  endocrine, 348–350
  female reproductive, 351–352, 353–355, 356–357
  gastrointestinal, 359–361, 363–365, 366–368, 370–372, 374–376, 378–380
  genitourinary, 381–383, 384–386, 387–389, 391–393
  musculoskeletal, 394–396, 398–401
  neonatal, 41, 45–46, 49–51
  nervous, 402–403, 404–406
  reports index, 10, 341
  respiratory, 408–411
  sense organ (eye), 413–415
Dissection, 14, 15, 348, 349
Distal, 167, 168, 179, 180, 181, 182, 203, 204, 223, 224, 273, 275, 279, 281, 298, 299, 384, 385
Diuresed, 278, 280
Diuretics, 132, 134

Diverticula, 220, 221
Diverticulitis, 363, 364
Dorsal, 233, 234
Dorsalis pedis, 344, 345
Dorsum, 167, 168, 335, 336
Drain, 374, 376
Draped, 264, 266
Duodenum, 115, 116, 287, 288, 294, 295, 374, 376
Dyazide, 356, 357
Dysphagia, 284, 285
Dysplasia, 25, 26
Dyspnea, 125, 126, 132, 133, 394, 395, 439
Dysrhythmia, 56, 60
Dysthymia, 52, 54
Dysuria, 391, 392

E

E. coli, 391, 393, 404, 405
Ecchymosis, 378, 379, 387, 388, 398, 399
Echocardiogram, 56, 58, 278, 280
Echogenicity, 209, 210
Ectopic pregnancy, 167, 168
Edema, 16, 17, 128, 129, 132, 134, 163, 164, 171, 173, 317, 318, 366, 367, 381, 383
EEG, 423
Effusion, 424
EKG, 47, 49
Electrocautery, 268, 269, 272, 274, 309, 310, 317, 318
Electrode, 423
Electrolyte, 363, 364
Elicited, 381, 383
Elongated, 427
Embolism, 147, 149
Embryonic/fetal development, 73f
Encroachment, 243, 244
Endarterectomy, 179, 180, 181, 182, 183, 184, 253, 254
Endometrial, 194, 195
Endometrial stripe, 71, 72
Endoscopic retrograde cholangiopancreatogram, 436
Endotracheal, 272, 274, 435
Endovaginally, 71, 72
Enterovirus, 47, 50
Epidermoid, 152, 153
Epididymis, 209, 210, 387, 389
Epididymitis, 387, 389
Epigastric, 272, 274
Epigastrium, 287, 288
Epinephrine, 264, 266, 307, 308, 333, 334
ER, 398, 399
ERCP, 374, 375
Erythema, 156, 157, 348, 349
Erythematous, 330, 331

Erythromycin, 18, 19
Esophagogastroduodenoscopy, 284, 285
Estrogen, 356, 357
Ethambutol, 408, 410
Etiology, 118, 119
ETOH, 344, 345
Excised, 314, 315, 321, 322
Excoriated fungating, 309, 310
Excrete, 203, 204
Exogenous, 273, 275
Exophytic, 152, 153
Exploratory, 366, 367
Exploratory laparotomy, 378, 380
Extensor tendon, 233, 234, 323, 324
External structure of the heart, 271f
Extramedullary, 404, 405
Extraocular, 171, 172
Extravasation, 203, 204, 206, 207, 438
Extubated, 335, 336, 404, 405

F

Facet, 243, 244
Fascia, 289, 290, 326, 327
Fascial, 321, 322
Female reproductive system, 70f, 193f
Femoral, 186, 187, 317, 318, 344, 345, 427
Femur, 326, 327
Fetal, 197, 198
Fetal circulation, 77f
Fibroadenoma, 428
Fibroadipose, 29, 30
Fibroid, 384, 385
Fibrotic, 115, 116
Fistula, 14, 15
5-FU, 137, 138
Flank, 159, 160
Flexion, 167, 168
Flexor retinaculum, 225, 226
Flexor tendon, 323, 324
Flexure, 220, 221
Fluoroscopic, 89, 90, 287, 288
Fluoroscopy, 262, 263, 264, 266
Focal, 95, 96, 425, 433
Foley, 366, 367, 413, 414
Foley catheter, 335, 336
Foramen of Winslow, 294, 295
Foramenal, 248, 249
Forceps, 268, 269
Formalin, 23, 24
Fornices, 37, 38
Fornix, 435
Fracture, 203, 204
Frontotemporal, 423
Frozen section, 356, 357
Fundal, 78, 79, 194, 195
Fundus, 132, 133
Fundi, 137, 138

Isordil, 404, 405
IV, 39, 41, 259, 260, 317, 318
IVP, 381, 383, 384, 385

J

Jaundice, 140, 141, 294, 295, 374, 375
Joint Commission on Accreditation of Healthcare Organizations (JCAHO), 5
Journal of the American Association for Medical Transcription (JAAMT). See American Association for Medical Transcription (AAMT)

K

Kidney structures, 110f
KUB, 384, 385

L

Lactated Ringer's, 262, 263
LAD, 272, 274
Laminectomy, 404, 405
Laparotomy, 363, 364, 366, 367, 368
Large intestine, 20f, 136f, 219f, 362f
Laryngectomy, 348, 349
Laryngoscopy, 330, 331
Lasix, 391, 392
Lateral, 78, 79, 301, 302, 304, 305, 317, 318, 323, 324, 326, 327, 335, 336
Lateral view of eyeball interior, 412f
Lateral view of external brain structure, 422f
Lateral view of the brain, 238f
Left ventricle dysfunction, 272, 274
Leiomyomatous, 384, 385
Leiomyosarcoma, 194, 195
Lesion, 233, 234, 309, 310
Lethargic, 128, 129
Leucovorin, 137, 138
LFT, 408, 410
LGA, 47, 49
Lidocaine, 264, 266, 301, 302, 307, 308, 317, 318, 323, 324, 333, 334
Ligated, 294, 295, 323, 324
Ligatures, 309, 310
Lipoma, 23, 24
Lipomatous, 321, 322
Lithotomy, 435
Lithotomy position, 434f
Lithotripsy, 391, 393
Liver and gallbladder, 373f
Liver, gallbladder, and pancreas, 94f, 139f, 292f, 358f
Location of the spleen in the abdominal cavity, 377f
Lumbar laminectomy, 402, 403
Lumbar myelogram, 404, 405
Lumbar spine, 248, 249

Lumen, 436
Lumpectomy, 356, 357
Lymph circulation, 316f
Lymph node, 317, 318
Lymphadenopathy, 65, 66, 99, 100, 118, 119, 137, 138, 171, 172, 314, 315
Lymphatic circulation, 114f
Lymphoma, 314, 315
Lysis, 363, 364

M

Magnevist, 437
Major arteries and veins of the body, 258f
Major arteries of the systemic circulation, 426f
Major veins of the body, 430f
Male reproductive system, 208f
Malecot catheter, 289, 290
Malleoli, 424
Malleolus, 424
Malposition of uterus, 419f
Mammogram, 163, 164
Mandibular, 398, 400
Marsupialized, 381, 383
Mastectomy, 304, 305
Maternal-fetal circulation, 81f
Mattress sutures, 279, 281
MB, 342, 343
Medial, 262, 263, 304, 305
Median, 272, 274
Mediastinal, 273, 275, 279, 283
Medical terms
    prefixes commonly used in, 445–446
    roots commonly used in, 448–449
    suffixes commonly used in, 446–447
Medical transcript, 1
Medical Transcription Industry Alliance (MTIA), 5
Medical transcriptionist (MT), 1
    career outlook, 5–6
    certified medical transcriptionist (CMT), 4
    certification, 4
    education, 4
    employment opportunities, 4
    transcription skills, 1
MediPort catheter, 264, 266
Medullary, 326, 327
mEq/L, 279, 282
Melanotic, 344, 346
Menarche, 356, 357
Meningioma, 404, 405
Mesenteric, 186, 187, 203, 204
Mesentery, 118, 119, 298, 299
Mesoappendicitis, 27, 28
Metacarpal, 223, 224
Metacarpals, 335, 336

Metastatic, 65, 66, 67, 68, 137, 138
Metastatic breast carcinoma, 353, 354
Metastatic carcinoma, 356, 357
Metatarsal, 323, 324
Methadone, 378, 379
Microcalcification, 428
Microlaryngoscopy, 330, 331
Midaxillary, 436
Midscapular, 333, 334
Mitral regurgitation, 132, 133
Mitral stenosis, 278, 280
Mitral valve, 278, 280
MLO, 425
MOM, 404, 406
Monoclonal, 31, 32
Morphology, 233, 234
Mortise, 424
MRI, 239, 240, 241, 242
MTB, 409, 410
Mucinous, 137, 138
Mucosal edema, 398, 399
Multinodulated, 147, 149
Musculature, 233, 234
Myelogram, 402, 403
Myocardial infarction, 125, 126, 128, 129, 342, 343, 353, 354
Myocardial ischemia, 439
Myocardium, 47, 50, 268, 269
Myocutaneous, 14, 15
Myoma, 194, 195, 199, 200

N

Nabothi cyst, 194, 195
Nasal cannula, 43, 45
Necrosis, 424
Necrotic, 37, 38, 144, 145, 301, 302, 307, 308, 409, 411
NED, 16, 17
Neoplasm, 102, 103, 436
Nephron, 211f, 390f
Nephrolithiasis, 159, 160
Nephrostomy, 438
Neuroleptic, 264, 266, 307, 308
NG tube, 363, 364
NICU, 39, 41
Nifedipine, 125, 126
Normocephalic, 140, 141, 366, 367, 378, 379
n.p.o., 47, 50, 128, 129, 363, 364
Nucleus pulposus, 402, 403

O

Oblique, 427, 428
Occiput, 309, 310
Occluded, 279, 281
Occlusion, 272, 274, 287, 288, 429
Omnipaque, 431
Oncovin, 253, 254
Opacification, 181, 182, 183, 184, 436

Pursestring suture, 289, 290
Purulent, 27, 28, 191, 192, 408, 410
PVCs, 132, 134
Pyelogram, 438
Pyelolithotomy, 217, 218
Pyelonephritis, 111, 112
Pyelovenous extravasation, 384, 385

Q
q.d., 404, 406
q8h, 47, 50
q.6h., 404, 405
Q's, 374, 375
Q-T, 47, 50
Quotation marks. *See* Punctuation
Qwave, 163, 165

R
RA, 264, 267
Radial, 344, 345
Radiating, 402, 403
Radiocarpal, 225, 226
Radioulnar, 225, 226
Rales, 132, 134
Ramus, 278, 280
RCA, 278, 280
Rectourethral, 14, 15
Rectus fascia, 294, 295
Rectus muscles, 289, 290
Reflux nephropathy, 111, 112
Renal, 163, 164, 203, 204, 217, 218, 431
Renal calculus, 95, 96, 391, 392
Resection, 298, 299
Residual, 436
Respiratory system, 250f
Retrograde, 279, 281, 294, 295
Retrograde IVP, 14, 15
Retroperitoneum, 65, 66, 92, 93, 99, 100, 102, 103, 203, 204, 206, 207
Retrorectal, 144, 145
Retroverted, 71, 72
Retroverted uterus, 420
Revascularization, 272, 274
Rifampin, 408, 410
Right bundle branch block, 374, 375
Right inguinal hernia, 378, 379
Rigors, 163, 164
Ringer's lactate, 317, 318
R/O, 31, 32
Rongeur, 323, 324

S
Sacral, 301, 302
Sacrectomy, 144, 145
Sacrococcygeal, 144, 145
Sacroiliac, 65, 66
Sacroiliac region, 356, 357
Sagittal, 225, 226, 239, 240, 241, 242, 243, 244, 424

Sagittal section of female breast, 162f, 303f
Sagittal section of the face and neck, 329f
Saline, 279, 281, 301, 302
Saphenous, 272, 274, 278, 280
Saphenous vein, 413, 414
Scalpel, 268, 269, 321, 322
Scapula, 335, 336, 394, 395
Scapular, 264, 266
Scarpa's fascia, 314, 315, 317, 318
Sclerae, 137, 138, 171, 172
Sclerotherapy, 201, 202
Scrotal, 381, 383
Scrotal hematoma, 387, 389
Scrotum, 381, 383
Sedated, 384, 385
Semicolon. *See* Punctuation
Sepsis, 39, 41
Sequential, 429
Serosa, 27, 28
Serous fluid, 268, 269
SFA, 344, 346
Sick sinus syndrome, 125, 126
SIDS, 47, 50
Sigmoid, 363, 364, 370, 371
Sigmoid colon, 220, 221
Singleton intrauterine gestation, 197, 198
Skeleton system, 325f
SMA-6, 128, 129, 394, 395, 413, 414
SONO, 71, 72, 82, 83, 92, 93
Sonograms of fetal development (22nd week), 85f
Sonography, 200, 300
S/P, 11, 12
Special procedures reports, 175
    cardiovascular, 179–180, 181–182, 183–184, 186–189
    endocrine, 191–192
    female reproductive, 194–195, 197–198, 199–200
    gastrointestinal, 201–202, 203–204, 206–207
    genitourinary, 209–210, 212–213, 214–215, 217–218
    hematic, 220–221
    musculoskeletal, 223–224, 225–226, 228–229, 231–232, 233–234
    nervous, 236–237, 239–240, 241–242, 243–244, 246–247, 248–249
    reports index, 177
    respiratory, 251–252, 253–254
Speciation, 409, 410
Sphincter, 159, 160
Spin echo, 231, 232, 243, 244
Spinal column, 143f, 227f
Spinous processes, 378, 379

Splenectomy, 378, 380
Splenic, 203, 204, 206, 207, 220, 221, 378, 380
Squamous, 152, 154
Squamous cell carcinoma, 309, 310
Stages of labor, 42f
Stasis, 287, 288
Status post, 370, 371, 398, 399
Stenosis, 179, 180, 183, 184, 248, 249, 272, 274, 287, 288, 427
Stents, 287, 288
Sternotomy, 272, 274
Streptomycin, 408, 410
Stricture, 436
ST-T, 128, 129
Styloid, 223, 224
Subacromial, 231, 232
Subcapsular, 203, 204, 206, 207
Subclavian, 259, 260, 264, 266
Subconjunctival hemorrhage, 398, 399
Subcortical, 437
Subcostal, 294, 295, 436
Subcutaneous, 167, 168, 233, 234, 262, 263, 264, 266, 268, 269, 289, 290, 321, 322
Subcuticular, 279, 282, 321, 322
Subcuticular sutures, 313f, 314, 315
Subdiaphragmatic, 191, 192
Subjugated, 56, 58
Submental, 171, 172
Subscapularis, 231, 232
Subserosal, 199, 200
Substernal, 125, 126
Superficial, 233, 234
Superior, 304, 305
Superior vena cava, 262, 263, 278, 281
Supine, 262, 263, 272, 274, 289, 290, 298, 299, 304, 305, 309, 310, 317, 318, 326, 327
Suppurative, 27, 28
Supraclavicular, 21, 22, 253, 254
Supraclavicular adenopathy, 147, 149, 152, 153
Suprapubic, 363, 364, 381, 383
Supraspinous, 231, 232
Supraventricular, 47, 49
Suture, 301, 302
Sutured, 435
Sutures, 323, 324
Swan-Ganz catheter, 278, 280, 298, 299
Symphysis, 99, 100, 102, 103, 115, 116, 118, 119
Syncope, 439
Synthroid, 348, 349
Systolic, 197, 198
Systolic blood pressure, 378, 379

System Requirements
- 100 MHz Pentium w/24 MB of RAM
- Windows(TM)95 or newer
- Sound card and speakers
- SVGA 24-bit color display
- 8 megabytes of free disk space

Microsoft® is a registered trademark and Windows™ and NT™ are trademarks of Microsoft Corporation.

Netware™ is a trademark of Novell, Inc.

Set-Up Instructions
1. Insert disk into CD ROM player
2. From the Start Menu, choose *RUN*
3. In the *Open* text box, enter **d: setup.exe** then click the *OK* button.(Substitute the letter of your CD ROM drive for **d:**)
4. Follow the installation prompts from there.

License Agreement for Delmar Learning, a division of Thomson Learning, Inc., Educational Software/Data

You the customer, and Delmar Learning, a division of Thomson Learning, Inc. incur certain benefits, rights, and obligations to each other when you open this package and use the software/data it contains. BE SURE YOU READ THE LICENSE AGREEMENT CAREFULLY, SINCE BY USING THE SOFTWARE/DATA YOU INDICATE YOU HAVE READ, UNDERSTOOD, AND ACCEPTED THE TERMS OF THIS AGREEMENT.

Your rights:

1. You enjoy a non-exclusive license to use the software/data on a single microcomputer in consideration for payment of the required license fee, (which may be included in the purchase price of an accompanying print component), or receipt of this software/data, and your acceptance of the terms and conditions of this agreement.
2. You acknowledge that you do not own the aforesaid software/data. You also acknowledge that the software/data is furnished "as is," and contains copyrighted and/or proprietary and confidential information of Delmar Learning, a division of Thomson Learning, Inc. or its licensors.

There are limitations on your rights:

1. You may not copy or print the software/data for any reason whatsoever, except to install it on a hard drive on a single microcomputer and to make one archival copy, unless copying or printing is expressly permitted in writing or statements recorded on the diskette(s).
2. You may not revise, translate, convert, disassemble or otherwise reverse engineer the software/data except that you may add to or rearrange any data recorded on the media as part of the normal use of the software/data.
3. You may not sell, license, lease, rent, loan or otherwise distribute or network the software/data except that you may give the software/data to a student or and instructor for use at school or, temporarily at home.

Should you fail to abide by the Copyright Law of the United States as it applies to this software/data your license to use it will become invalid. You agree to erase or otherwise destroy the software/data immediately after receiving note of termination of this agreement for violation of its provisions from Delmar Learning.

Delmar Learning, a division of Thomson Learning, Inc gives you a LIMITED WARRANTY covering the enclosed software/data. The LIMITED WARRANTY follows this License.

This license is the entire agreement between you and Delmar Learning, a division of Thomson Learning, Inc. interpreted and enforced under New York law.

LIMITED WARRANTY

Delmar Learning, a division of Thomson Learning, Inc. warrants to the original licensee/purchaser of this copy of microcomputer software/data and the media on which it is recorded that the media will be free from defects in material and workmanship for ninety (90) days from the date of original purchase. All implied warranties are limited in duration to this ninety (90) day period. THEREAFTER, ANY IMPLIED WARRANTIES, INCLUDING IMPLIED WARRANTIES OF MERCHANTABILITY AND FITNESS FOR A PARTICULAR PURPOSE, ARE EXCLUDED. THIS WARRANTY IS IN LIEU OF ALL OTHER WARRANTIES, WHETHER ORAL OR WRITTEN, EXPRESS OR IMPLIED.

If you believe the media is defective please return it during the ninety day period to the address shown below. Defective media will be replaced without charge provided that it has not been subjected to misuse or damage.

This warranty does not extend to the software or information recorded on the media. The software and information are provided "AS IS." Any statements made about the utility of the software or information are not to be considered as express or implied warranties.

Limitation of liability: Our liability to you for any losses shall be limited to direct damages, and shall not exceed the amount you paid for the software. In no event will we be liable to you for any indirect, special, incidental, or consequential damages (including loss of profits) even if we have been advised of the possibility of such damages.

Some states do not allow the exclusion or limitation of incidental or consequential damages, or limitations on the duration of implied warranties, so the above limitation or exclusion may not apply to you. This warranty gives you specific legal rights, and you may also have other rights which vary from state to state. Address all correspondence to: Delmar Learning, a division of Thomson Learning, Inc., 5 Maxwell Drive, P.O. Box 8007, Clifton Park, NY 12065–8007. Attention: Technology Department.